This book is dedicated to you and your healing.

~~~~~~~

Writing to Heal

A Pandemic Journey to Healing

Anthony Fleg MD, MPH

ISBN 979-8-44-7397685

Published by Community Publishing
Albuquerque, New Mexico

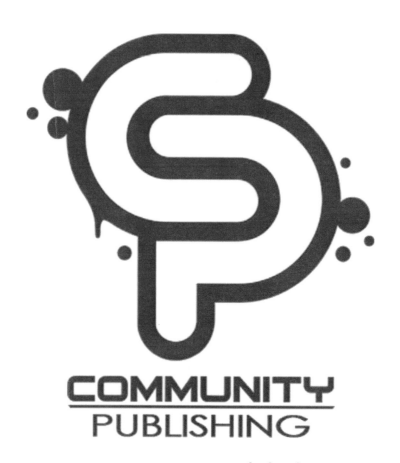

COMMUNITY PUBLISHING

wwwcommunitypublishing.org
info@communitypublishing.org

Table of Contents

1. Prologue by Hakim Bellamy   I

2. Foreword by David Rakel   II

3. Welcome to Writing to Heal   III

4. 2020 Timeline   IV

5. A Gratitude Perspective on Coronavirus   1

6. The Superpower of Being Present   3

7. Turning North to Get South   5

8. Wind, Our Teacher   7

9. Job Description: Exhaustion   10

10. Service: Antidote to Fear   12

11. In Memory of Chei Bahe Manybeads   15

12. The Oxygen Cycle   18

13. Corona – Tha Verse   20

14. The Shoe-less Hike   23

15. When Life Gives You Lemons…Fermentation Begins   25

16. Flow With It   27

17. White supremacy: Time to Cure the Disease   29

18. Strawberry Wisdom   32

19. "There is still Normal" vs. "Nothing is Normal"   34

20. Love for Community - The Emelia Pino story   37

21. Celebrating Inter-Dependence This July 4th!   39

22. I Am Sorry   41

23. Kindness (aka Love for Community Part 2: The Nehemiah Cionelo Story)   44

24. Renewal   47

25. Of Tree Lines and Tolerance   50

26. In the Dark No More   52

27. Going to a Special Place   54

28. Sacred Play and Imaginary Escapes   56

29. Connection   59

30. Signs of Change   61

31. The Ever-Present Presence of the Present   64

32. Gháájí': New Year, New You   66

33. Bass and Treble   67

34. Mask Up!   69

35. Explosion   71

36. Jump!   73

37. A Vision for Undoing Racism + Achieving Equity in Health   75

38. Writing to Heal: The 45-Word Edition   77

39. Bowls into Cabinets   79

40. Gratitude   81

41. Drift   85

42. Vaccinating Despair, Injecting Hope   86

43. Shepherd's Journey   88

44. Gratitude and Acknowledgments   v

45. About the Author   vi

46. About the Cover Art   vii

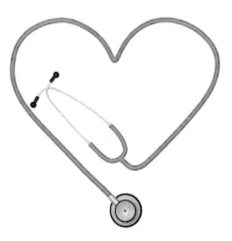

Prologue

Dr. Anthony Fleg is my brother. And like any good sibling (be they by birth, blood, basketball or bond), he has a way of getting me to do things I do not want to do. Like run. He is good at getting people of all walks of life to do the very thing they dreaded in grade school gym class. He does it with a smile. He does it with no judgment. He does it out of a cherubic desire to see you surprise yourself. The enthusiasm he brings to those moments of achievement when you genuinely surprise yourself rivals the "wow" factor that a child experiences on Christmas morning. It is infectious. Perhaps that's a poor choice of words with respect to some of the thematic content herein, but in a fateful twist of irony … it is *also* medicine.

What happens when well-being is contagious?

What happens when gratitude is contagious?

What happens when service is contagious?

What happens when love is contagious?

It's hard to imagine a world where positivity is contagious at the current moment in time. However, it is precisely that imagination that *Writing to Heal* prescribes. Physicians are experts at getting us to do things we don't want to do … that are good for us. Things like having patience. Things like getting more rest. Things like eating more and drinking less (unless it's water, drink more water). Things like running. Thinks like writing and reading (the kind that doesn't require a screen). Things like being grateful, like breathing, like sitting still.

Mostly, my brother Anthony reminds me to make time to play. For many "grown ups" *play* is their least favorite four-letter word. Or maybe that's least frequent? Or rather least familiar? Rhymes with *pray*. This "playbook" is a kind of manual to kick-start your practice of radical imagination, the kind that creates a world (or word) where all things good are contagious.
Thanks in advance ... for playing along.

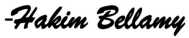

Albuquerque's Inaugural Poet Laureate
www.beyondpoetryink.com

Foreword

Kathy was trying to get pregnant for over a year. As her family physician, I was honored to be invited into the context of her life and she felt comfortable sharing stories of her past. She told me of an assault that she had been holding inside herself for many years and she was finding it difficult to forgive the aggressor.

After doing all the tests for infertility and finding nothing of concern, we wondered if that event could be related to her body's resistance to accepting a new life. We didn't know the answer, but Kathy was willing to explore. I asked that she write a letter to her assailant, letting the pain from her body flow onto the paper. She was instructed to write down her deepest emotions, not holding back.

She then sealed the letter in an envelope and lit it on fire. As the wind carried the smoke away, her internalized suffering went with it. Twelve months later, I delivered her first child.

Disease loves stagnation. Healing requires movement and flow. When I reflect on what Anthony Fleg has taught me, flow and connection ring true. He is an artist in connecting people through his kind heart, infectious positive spirit and beautiful reflections. And through this connection, flow happens.

The writings in this book are a beautiful example of connecting to the authentic truth that is all around us, even when it is difficult to see during COVID times. It encourages us to pick up a journal and use our own experiences to write, inviting new life into the world.

Dave Rakel, M.D.

Professor and Chair, University of Wisconsin
Dept. of Family Medicine and Community Health

Welcome to Writing to Heal

My name is Anthony Fleg and like you, I have tried to make sense of life during COVID-19 one day at a time.

The pandemic has inspired me to write, and more specifically *Writing to Heal*.

It all began with a moment at the dinner table 10 days into the pandemic where I asked the question of my children, "What do you think this moment is here to teach us?"

My oldest daughter replied immediately. "I think it is here to teach us to be grateful for our health."

I wrote a piece inspired by this simple answer that Wednesday, and after a few weeks of doing this every Wednesday night, it became a blog and part of my way of healing and coping with pandemic living.

I would create time to sit and pen a piece based on what comes to me. Thoughtful pieces but not necessarily thought out – the energy is spontaneous, spiritual, and very much about learning and healing from this moment.

While the pandemic serves as a backdrop for Writing to Heal, I have written in the moment about what I think needs to be written on: George Floyd's murder, the arrival of the COVID vaccine, and more recently, the struggle that is the 3rd wave.

I think the short pieces in Writing to Heal will give both a time capsule from the pandemic, while also remaining pertinent far beyond the pandemic.

I hope this book will bring healing to you in your journey.

I look forward to healing together.

In health,

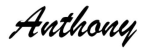

At the end of most pieces, there is an action/reflection for you to take the piece and make it useful for you and your journey.

You are invited to share your thoughts on the Writing to Heal blog (writingtoheal1.blogspot.com) or on social media (instagram.com/writing_to_heal_book/)

2020 Timeline

March 11: The World Health Organization declares the Coronavirus outbreak a pandemic.

March 11 and 12: The NBA, NHL, MLB, NFL and NCAA all suspend their sports seasons. The NCAA Indoor Track Championships, slated for Albuquerque, are canceled hours before the start of competition.

March 13: Breonna Taylor is murdered in Louisville, KY.

March 19: NM Businesses ordered to close, including malls, movie theaters, health clubs and spas.

March 24: NM issues first stay-at-home order and discourages gatherings of five or more people. All nonessential businesses are ordered to close.

March 25: First COVID-19 related death in NM.

March 26: Global Coronavirus cases top 500,000. The U.S. reaches 1,000 COVID deaths.

March 27: NM Public Education Dept. orders all schools to cancel in-person learning.

March 31: New York passes 75,000 Coronavirus case, half of the U.S. total. U.S. COVID deaths reach 3,000. Seventy percent of the U.S. population is under lockdown.

April 3: The CDC recommends that everyone consider wearing cloth or fabric face masks in public.

Late April: U.S. death toll from COVID-19 surpasses 50,000 while worldwide cases surpass 3 million.

May: NM's Indigenous communities continue to be disproportionately affected by COVID. Representing 10% of the state's population, Indigenous communities account for 58% of NM's COVID cases as of late May.

May 7: Gregory and Travis McMichael are charged with murder in the death of Ahmaud Arbery 2/23/20 in Georgia.

May 11: NM opens up COVID-19 testing to all New Mexicans.

May 16: Phase 1 of reopening; New Mexicans are ordered to wear a mask in all public spaces.

May 25: George Floyd is murdered in Minneapolis, MN.

May 28: A state of emergency is declared in Minneapolis-St. Paul as protests over the death of George Floyd and racial injustice spread nationwide.

June: Balloon Fiesta and State Fair, two of NM's biggest annual events, are canceled.

June 30: Mississippi retires the official state flag - the last state flag incorporating the Confederate flag.

July 30: NBA season resumes in the NBA "bubble" in Orlando.

August/September: Wildfires rage through California and Oregon.

August 23: Protests break out in Kenosha, Wis., after the shooting of 29-year-old Jacob Blake by a police officer.

August 29: NM restaurants allowed to resume indoor dining at 25% capacity. Other restrictions are loosened in this order.

Sept. 22: The death toll of the pandemic in the United States passes 200,000.

October: The 2nd Wave of COVID-19 begins.

Nov 9-16: Pfizer and Moderna release data showing their COVID-19 vaccines to be 90% effective.

November 16: NM issues a two-week lock down amidst 2nd wave a rising cases/hospitalization.

December: In the midst of the 2nd Wave, many hospitals and ICUs are over 100% capacity.

December 2: NM implements "Red, Yellow, Green" system for loosening restrictions.

Dec. 14: The first COVID-19 vaccinations start in the United States.

Dec. 27: Vaccine distribution widens in NM beyond front-line workers.

Jan 26, 2021: New Mexico schools given green-light to start hybrid mode.

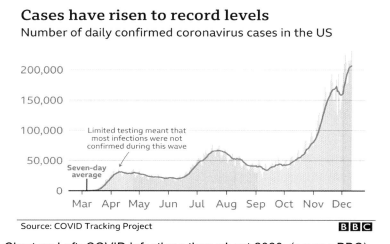

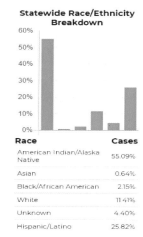

Chart on Left: COVID infections throughout 2020. (source BBC)

Chart on Right: Disproportionate COVID infections in New Mexico's Indigenous communities as of June 2020. (source NM DOH)

A Gratitude Perspective on Coronavirus

I often turn to my children when facing life's vexing moments. So I did just that. "Kiddos, what do you think Coronavirus is here to teach us?"

My 11 year-old spoke first, "To be thankful for our health."

Gratitude, huh?

I stepped back from this moment and wonder if she is on to something.

Working as a physician and educator at the University of New Mexico (UNM and having spent the better part of the last days thinking about the implications of COVID-19 for our New Mexico population down to the level of patients and students, I am thankful for this moment.

If you will allow, I would like to infuse some Coronavirus-induced gratitude into the moment in which we find ourselves.

First, a time to see more clearly the importance of the people and communities that sustain us. Reflect on this when (likely today…again! your workplace huddles together to discuss COVID-19 precautions and procedures. It is so easy to work around great people and, distracted by the work to be done, forget to appreciate those doing the work. Reflect on it, but don't stop there – tell the beautiful people around you how much you value them. I can't leave this topic without thinking of the epidemic of loneliness that afflicts our society that claims to be so technologically connected - take a moment to notice the neighbor, classmate, work colleague who do not have community and invite them into yours.

Second, in a world eternally on fast forward, truncated to 140 character messages, Coronavirus gives us a moment to pause, breathe deep, slow down, dig deeper. Self care – increase the dose! Story time with your children – increase the dose! Prayer, exercise and other ways that you connect with yourself and things larger than you – increase the dose! Start today with the birds and trees outside your house and office that greet you only to have you rush past without a nod or smile. Continue with the food you eat – take a moment to slow down and be mindful of how this food got to your plate. Consume accordingly. Consider this next few weeks an extended snow day, an invitation to slow down to a healthier speed of living than our usual. And since angst and anxiety are among us, spreading like the virus itself, your work to slow down and breathe deep will be good medicine.

Last, a very simple ask of myself and all of us, returning to my daughter's advice – gratitude. Make a point today to express gratitude. If necessary, use words. Make your living something the poets and prophets speak of, gratitude in your heart and hands (washed frequently, of course). In the 100,000 heartbeats, 20,000 breaths, and the 86,400 seconds that make today, take a few heartbeats, breaths, and seconds to give thanks. Increase dose steadily.

The test question for my students would be simple:

"Coronavirus – curse or blessing?"

You get to decide today what answer to choose!

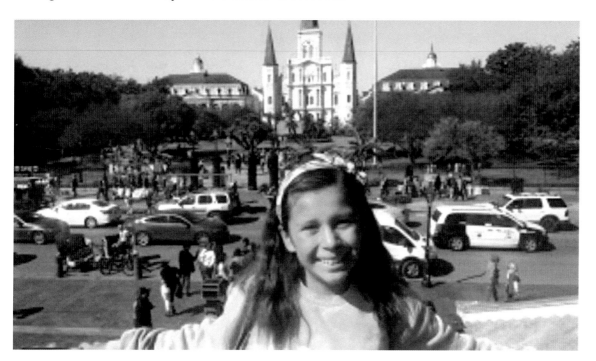

Action/Reflection:

Write down 3 things you are grateful for in this moment.

Repeat this 2-3 more times today. Each time, simply pause and write down 3 things you are grateful for in that moment.

Take your "gratitude list" of the words from above and let them guide a piece on gratitude.

The Superpower of Being Present

I turned to my 2-year old daughter with a simple ask:
"Can you worry about tomorrow for me?"

Blank stare.

"All I am asking is that you worry about tomorrow.
Just follow the lead of us adults who make it look easy.
Now, can you do that for daddy? (Don't you know about
the latest case of Coronavirus?)"

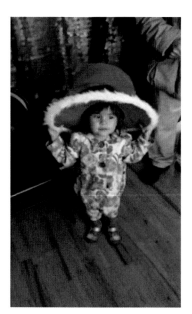

Blank stare.

Now, a quick question for all of us – how much of each day do
we spend worrying about the future, particularly as it relates
to Coronavirus? How much time is our mind spent on
tomorrow, next week, April, June, etc.?

I would have gotten a similar blank stare if I were to demand
that my daughter worry about what happened yesterday, last week, or 30 minutes ago.

Think of the children in your life, in your family. Bring their presence to mind and imagine
what a wonderful superpower they possess: **an inability to live anywhere but the
present. Their superpower is living in the moment.**

This moment, the COVID-19 chapter of our world and of our lives, implores us to be more
like our children in this regard.

Being present is a wonderful thing. It relieves stress caused by focusing on failures of the
past and worries of the future. Both realms are un-reachable, largely un-changeable. But
at the same time, they both entice and tease our minds such that we often find ourselves
everywhere but in the moment as we focus on changing what has already passed or what
may (or may not) come to be.

Living as our children model so well, in the moment, has an immediate influence on our
health and wellness. Tuning out the constant barrage of news about Coronavirus and
tuning into what is before you will bring calm, serenity, and a sense that all is okay. It will
allow you to enjoy the moment, the small pleasures our senses offer us, things that pass
us by when we are lost somewhere else on the time continuum. The touch of an elder,
the smell of a blossoming fruit tree, the way the wind feels against our cheek - open up to
the present and it is all there for you.

Just ask the 2 -year olds.

In this time where we more than ever need to be there for family, friends, neighbors, co-workers and our larger community, there is no more important place to start than to work on being more present. When that phone call comes, frantic and worried voice on the other end, they need a "you" that is grounded in what *is*. Not what *was*. Not what might come to be. But grounded in what *is* at that moment.

A simple ask for today – let's re-kindle that superpower of our children. Let us put aside the constant news feeds and social media posts about a world with no TP, all of it distractions from the gift that is the present. Let us be more mindful to gently steer the thought train back to the moment when it starts to take us elsewhere.

I imagine coming to my toddler for advice, and instead of blank stare, this is what I would hear:

"Dad, watch yourself breathing. Pay attention to the sensation of "being". Fall in love with the moment you are in, because you won't have it back."

"Now, dad, can you dig in the dirt with me? Play, that's my other superpower."

Action/Reflection:

Step back from what you are doing, take a few deep breaths and let your mind slow. Close your eyes if that seems natural. Breathe in the present. Notice what you smell, what you hear, what you feel. Take as long as you want. Repeat a few more times today.

Take time today to write about the experience of breathing in the present.

Turning North to Get South

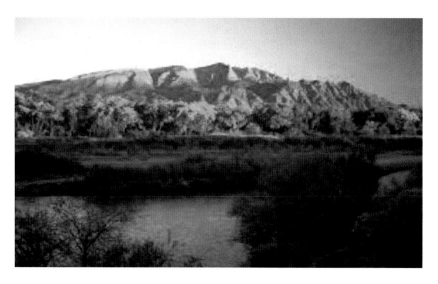

In running, I find healing and meaning in some of their purest forms. I have always thought that I could write a "how-to" guide on life just from the lessons learned while flying over the trails.

No technology to track my steps or miles, no fancy gear, nothing to sync my data to show the rest of the world *(if a tree falls in a forest and it is not captured on social media, did it really happen? The answer my millennial students would give is a "What tree? What forest?".*

So, feeling a bit drained from a long week, I laced up my shoes and headed to the strong medicine of the Sandia Mountains for three hours of play.

I was about an hour into the run when I got directions from a friend I happened to pass on the trail.

"It's going to look like you are going the wrong direction, heading north, but that trail will take you home to the south."

From 6 feet away I panted "Thanks, brother." I climbed further into my playground, trying to accept that heading north was actually going to get me south.

In our current moment, there is comfort we can find in having someone to guide us.

Reflect on all of the messages you received in the last 48 hours from authorities about new restrictions and updated procedures related to coronavirus, all of them asking us to turn north, just to make it to the south. Beyond feeling inundated and overwhelmed, perfectly normal responses, do you remember feeling a sense of relief that someone was guiding your way?

Did you take a moment to think about what it means for our communities and larger society that we are able to work for the collective good in a way that we rarely see?

When those emails, "alert texts" and newsflashes come across your screens today, pause, breathe deep and give thanks for the CDCs, the DOHs, the frontline healthcare workers of the world who are there to protect and guide us. Yes, we are all being asked to turn north with a promise that it will be our best way to make it south safely. Again, find comfort that someone is there to guide your/our path. Allow yourself to trust that advice.

Well, being both stubborn and directionally-challenged, a few hours after that encounter, I found myself nowhere near my starting point and heading south, climbing higher and higher. You would have thought that the patches of snow and glimpses of the ridge that signaled the top of the mountain would have kind of, sort of told me I might want to re-evaluate my current path since I needed to end up about 3,000 feet lower than my elevation at that moment. (Perfectly okay to laugh here).

"I am heading south so I must be going the right way!" I told myself over and over. Our lives are the route. The map in our head tells us the only way to turn is south, blinding us from seeing that we clearly headed the wrong way.

Maybe COVID-19 (or "Mr. 19" as one of my patient's nicknamed it) is the turn to the north that will get us where we are meant to go???? With some bumps and tests of faith along the way, but maybe it is getting us "home" despite our feeling that it is taking us the wrong way.

My friends, "Mr. 19" has turned us north.

Let's accept it.

Let's embrace it.

Find joy in the path ahead.

Be an active part of it getting yourself "home" in a way that, like a long run, leaves us replenished and renewed even if exhausted.

P.S. In case you are worrying that I am writing this stranded in the mountains, I did make it to the car, just under the 6-hour mark. Replenished, renewed, exhausted. The blessing was not the finish line, but the journey north that it took to get there.

Action/Reflection:
When today brings you to a turn that your instinct is the wrong way, stop before you reject it. Consider "turning north" even if your plan was to go south in that moment.

Write about a time when you turned north just to get south, reflecting on what you learned from that moment.

Wind, Our Teacher

Wind.

It seems to be ever-present in the early spring days of New Mexico.
Heavy wind, blowing day after day can be aggravating. One scientific theory behind this is that wind disrupts our sense of equilibrium. There is even a condition – ancraophobia – that is an extreme fear of wind.

We could complain about the strong gusts that will likely greet us today (again, intent on blowing us off our feet, ruining our hair.

But you wouldn't be reading this if that were you.

What is the wind is trying to teach us in this pandemic moment?

Part 1: Indigenous wisdom on the wind

Our Indigenous traditions are quite clear that wind is a powerful way to cleanse what

needs to be blown away.

A Dine' colleague shares "When you pray and the wind shows its presence, the Holy Ones are with you."

Karen Waconda-Lewis (Isleta/Laguna relates, "Wind is the sacred Air Element. Air Element comes to us at the first breath. In spring, Air Element is most active after winter when it sleeps. Just like birth."

CC Alonso de Franklin (Mexica/Lipan Apache adds, *Ehecatl* is the God of the wind, part of fertility. We are not to be afraid of the wind because it cleanses, it takes away what is no longer needed. She continues in describing *Ehecatl*, "It lacks physical form and is an energy that cannot be pinned down. We have to flow with it."

So much wisdom in those interpretations.

Let me translate this into a wind meditation we can all practice today.
Greet the wind, turning into the wind with arms outstretched to your sides. Flow with it. Take a moment here – how good and freeing it is to greet the wind that we often spend so much energy resisting.

Feel the Air Element as it passes between fingers, brushes against face. Feel its breath, its embrace.

Now, let it do the work of cleansing. Ehacatl, wipe away that which does not serve me and humankind to live to our truest self."Name things needing to be swept away if that is meaningful for you.

Take as much time as you need.

Close with gratitude in your own way, language, and tradition.

Part 2: Bike-ride wisdom on the wind

I had a hard-to-explain moment with the wind last week.

I had convinced my two oldest children to bike a long distance with me, and we headed north. The wind was heavy and at our backs.

"Dad, this feels so easy. There is no wind today."

Hmmm…How do I explain to them that when wind is pushing us we often don't appreciate its presence? How do I explain why we only notice it when it is a headwind in our face?

The tailwind is all that we take for granted – food, shelter, safety, love, family, community. It is privilege – the tailwind that accompanies Whiteness, being male, being heterosexual, speaking English fluently, having U.S. Citizenship, formal education, wealth, etc. Tailwinds blow many of us in the direction of success, leading to a sense of "This feels so easy." Those with that heavy tailwind pushing them often wonder why others are struggling to achieve.

Even as we mature, it is a challenge to see the way the winds blow us forward.

We are now in a global moment where my kids were when we turned 180 degrees and began to head home, to the south. Heavy, gusting, unrelenting wind in our face.

"Dad, where did this wind come from?"

This headwind we find ourselves in gives us chances to recognize the blessings the *tailwind life* has granted us all along. Start with the simple joys of being around others at a park, at a play, at the store, even in the waiting room of MVD or a dentist's office – do you appreciate these just a bit more in the headwind of COVID-19? Take a moment to reflect on your own privilege and how it blows doors open that for others shut in their face.

The headwind makes us push a bit harder for things we have taken for granted.

In the case of the bike ride, it was the way back that was going to reveal my children's fortitude and resilience.

Complain, they did. (luckily for daddy, the wind was strong enough that I could not make out much of what they were saying.....shhhh, don't tell them).

But it was the way back, not the way out, that strengthened them for the next ride. In the strong headwinds of life, the blessings lie.

As we turn the corner into April, we have just barely made the 180 degree turn into the Coronavirus wind.

There will be tough moments on this ride home, and we might even find ourselves struggling, wondering if we will make it.

Don't focus right now on making it out of this headwind, making it home. The blessing is in embracing the wind, flowing with it, learning from it as it cleanses us on the way.

Thank you, wind.

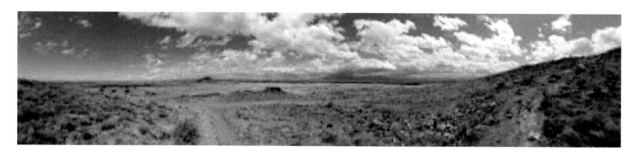

Picture taken while facing/embracing strong westerly winds on a March day
from the Volcanoes National Monument west of Albuquerque.

Action/Reflection:

Try the wind meditation from this piece today. If the weather gives you wind, try it outside. Otherwise, imagine facing into the wind as you try it. Or, do the meditation with focus on a wind"challenge that you are facing in life.

Reflect on the tailwind in your life. Write about it.

Job Description: Exhaustion

It has been 5 weeks, 5 Wednesday nights. The ritual of sitting with blank piece of electronic paper and making something happen. Building community around this simple act of writing. I am thankful.

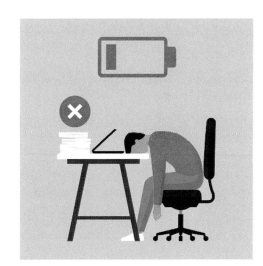

While it has all been focused on healing in this moment, I have avoided some of the day-to-day struggles that all of us face in this "new normal" of Zoom-living, cabin fever disequilibrium.

But, I have heard it too many times in the last week to ignore.

"I feel like my work is asking way too much of me. I am working harder than ever, it seems. **I am exhausted.**"

A family physician myself, I am reduced to seeing patients by phone visits. The volume is low compared to normal, yet I too share in that exhaustion.

Let us explore and understand the exhaustion together for a moment. First, we must travel to a different world than our current one. Let us time travel far back, to the *The World of February 2020*.

Remember that world? You were buying your spring concert tickets, signing the kids up for baseball and soccer leagues? You were hugging people and should anyone keep 6 feet apart from you, you would have taken it as an insult. Crazy, huh? Okay, so traveling back to *The World of February 2020*, you get a job offer that reads as follows:

"Great job, perfect for the extremely flexible. Rules, protocols, and responsibilities will change daily. Emails with a tone of "we might need to *really* start panicking now" will fly at you every 3-5 minutes. You will have to work with people without being in the room with people, with no drop in your efficiency. You must quickly master something called Zoom and develop *Zoom* skills such as "how to raise your hand" and "picking a background picture" on this technology. As an added perk to this job, you may have to be a full-time school teacher simultaneously while you work for us. Oh, one more thing - your time off from work will involve confinement in the home, so that work will become the majority of socialization in your weekly routine."

Yikes! Raise your hand if you would sign up for that job. (No need to use *Zoom* for this).

Imagine how quickly the labor unions of *The World of February 2020* would reject this! Medical diagnosis in *The World of February 2020* would be *Meshuggah*, Yiddish for CRAZY!

A moment to sigh together.

A chance to understand together the fatigue that we are feeling.
On some levels, most of us are doing less work, producing less in our time at work. But the exhaustion is about the work of adapting, bending, contorting ourselves each day, each week, over and over to a new way of being, both in the 9 to 5 and the rest of our lives is CRAZY! Exhausting!

Three prescriptions for our collective exhaustion – appreciate, structure, and laughter.

Appreciate: Take time today to appreciate the work you have done to adapt to a new world that we would have laughed at just 30 days ago or in *The World of February 2020*. Take arms forward and wrap them around upper torso for a tight self-hug. Affirmation that this current world is exhausting. Patience with self, reminding that fatigue is inevitable with the job description and life disequilibrium we have been handed. Replace resisting the exhaustion with working to accept it.

Structure: Take a piece of electronic or tree-derived paper and draw out your schedule for today and the following two days. Step back and take a look at what your current schedule/structure looks like. Are there simple things that you can change that would relieve cognitive load? Now that most are working from home, have you set rules about how to set a firm end to the work-day, a point beyond which calls and emails are left for the following day? Is there structure for fun and play included in your schedule? Make changes as needed!

Laughter: It might be one of our best medicines in all of this. Seriously, can we just laugh for a moment at what our current *job description* and *life description* has evolved into? Imagine us all around a campfire (not even 6 feet apart from one another!) in *The World of February 2020* enjoying a hearty laugh as we ready the job description above. Laugh and keep laughing! Best results when done with others.
My brothers and sisters in exhaustion, as the saying goes, "When the *The World of February 2020* laughs at you, you join in the laughter!"

Action/Reflection:

Make a mental note of the things you do today that you would never have done in *The World of February 2020*. Feel free to smile/laugh as you create this list.

Write a piece from the vantage point of you in *The World of February 2020* observing what you did today. Have fun with this one.

Service to Others: Antidote for Fear

It started with a trip to the zoo. The gorilla exhibit, to be exact.

Our youngest daughter Sihasin, meaning "to have hope" in Navajo, was quite afraid of these creatures. They looked and acted just a bit too much like humans. Giraffes – beautiful and tall. Hippos – wet and splashy. Both intimidating in their own right, but it was the human-ness of the gorillas that got to her.

I had an idea.

"Sihasin, can you hold my hand please? I am scared of these gorillas. Please."
She turned to me and forgot her own fright, reached for my hand, and proceeded to gently walk me past the gorillas.

"Dad, it's okay. Don't be scared."

As the pandemic settles in, all of us are scared. All of us see the gorilla and want to know how to overcome the fear it causes. (Trying hard to avoid cliché mention of the 800lb… whew…almost!)

I would say, on behalf of Sihasin who could not be here tonight due to "bedtime rules", that reaching out to hold someone's hand is the best antidote we can find.
There is so much we can do to serve others, to hold their hand right now - delivering food boxes, sewing masks, and spreading kindness are becoming infectious in an incredible way.

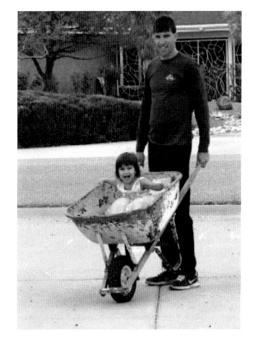

What happens when we turn the TV and news off, turning our hands and heart into a more positive direction. For you. For your neighbor. For those in dire need.

Back to Sihasin.

We found that this technique worked quite well with her in many situations. Loud noises from trucks, vacuum cleaners and the like really rattle her. But without fail, once we show her our fear of that same item, she loses all sense of fright and goes into helping mode.

Think for a moment I bet you have witnessed in your own self a moment that illustrates this principle in your own life.

Maybe even a moment in the last week, as this pandemic has given us lots of gorilla exhibit moments. For the parents and grandparents, maybe you have seen this technique work with your little ones.

But there was a moment that stunned me, reminding me the innate wisdom our little ones have.

We were in a public place, which for a 2-year old immediately sets off an alarm located in the bladder.

"Daddy, I need to go potty," she wiggled and wriggled.

Off to the potty we went. Uh-oh. Vacuum cleaner. A loud one.

The ritual began – her expressing fear, daddy expressing my own fear. Sihasin reaching for my hand, pulling me toward the bathroom.

But on the way out, she did something brand new. Remember that the two minutes in the bathroom is an eternity for a little mind. So, I prepared to replay the same ritual as we got done washing our hands.

Instead, before I said anything, as we left the bathroom she grabs my hand and rushes me past the still loud, obnoxious, threatening vacuum cleaner.

Dad, it's okay. Don't be scared."

She had made the connection without me having to prompt her. She didn't even ask if I was scared. It didn't matter. What she had figured out for herself was that the best way to overcome her fear was to focus on being there for me.

Whether gorilla or vacuum cleaner analogy works better for you, put this into action today around your fears in this moment and when life returns to normal. Find someone whose hand you will hold, knowing it is a win-win proposition. Symbiosis in its simplest form.

Some of us will need some prompting, for instance an email/text/voicemail of desperation that becomes the outstretched hand that we will reach to grab. Or maybe, like Sihasin, we can go one step further, reaching out our hands, trusting that someone else will be there to grab on.

In a non-pandemic moment, the question might be "What do I get out of this"and "Whose hand am I about to touch?" and "What if there is no hand there at all." Often, this line of questions convinces us not to reach hand out at all.

Our current situation, with a globe unified in its suffering, helps us overcome those questions, helping us see how and who we can be, now and always. This moment teaches us that the hand that meets ours will lead both to a better place.

Translated to Sihasin's world: to the hippos and giraffes.

Action/Reflection:

When you see a "gorilla" today, reach out to serve someone else instead of focusing on the gorilla.

Write about what happened when you did the above!

In Memory of Cheii Bahe Manybeads, 6.20.1925 - 4.4.2020

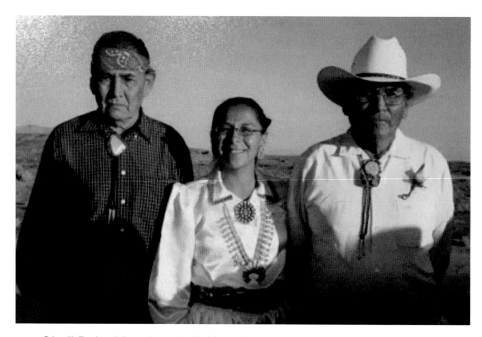

Cheii Bahe Manybeads (left) with his brother Cheii Eddie (right) with Shannon on our wedding day.

Grandpa

Uncle

Brother

Cheii

Hatałii

Our grandpa, 95 years this June,

Has crossed over to next world, the virus ushering him forward

Loving embrace still felt

Laughter echoing

Learning carried on by all he touched

Leaving us to follow his lead

> *How to serve others*
>
> *How to master the simple life*
>
> *How to cultivate our medicine*

From my wife Shannon, as she remembers her grandfather:

'Cheii Bahe Manybeads was a man that was never a great uncle, or just my *Cheii* (maternal grandfather) Eddie's brother.

He was my *Cheii,* and I am very fortunate to have known him for all these years. I probably met him in my youth but don't remember. But I never knew my *Cheii* Eddie had a brother, and I had an aunts and uncles from that relationship. I was fortunate to rekindle the relationship when I was in high school.

My *Cheii* Bahe was always considered to be very intelligent. My mother explained that he was one who finished school, learning how to speak and read not only in English but *Diné* too! He was one of my inspirations for continuing school, and keeping my traditional perspective in *Diné* . He was also one I think of as being really funny, while being so serious at the same time. When my mother and I visited him and his wife, he would like to tell stories, and show his new inventions to something he made. He also enjoyed when we brought my *Cheii* Eddie and *Masan* i Mae to visit. But he really liked it when his brother Eddie visited them. I would just listen to them talk about the things they had done 30 years ago, as if it just happened the day before.

Their relationship reminded me of how love and faith keep a friendship alive. They taught that each day should not be taken for granted. They taught me life is precious, they taught me to respect all are our relations. They taught me, to just be me, no matter what changed around me. I trusted, honored, respected, and loved these two gentlemen.

When it can time for me to marry, my *Cheii* Bahe is one gentleman I wanted to be involved with the *Diné* marriage ceremony. And so, I asked him if he could do the honors of provide the medicine for our marriage. At first, he was hesitant because like all *Diné* grandfathers he was stingy. He was wondering, "Who is this guy that wants to marry my granddaughter? Is he worthy? How much is he going to give me?"

He gave me a hard time, asking with a smile, "Is this the guy?" He made me laugh so much, and I kept telling him "Yes!" I had to ask my aunt to help get him to say "yes" to carrying out the ceremony, like I was asking *him* to marry me. He eventually gave in, leading the blessing of walking me into my Diné marriage with my husband and both of our families.

Ahéhee' (thank you) for giving the blessing of marriage.
Cheii was more than an *Hataɬii* (Medicine Man).

He *was* the medicine.

Hózhó nahásdlíí' (May beauty be restored).
Hózhó náhásdlíí' (May beauty be restored).
Hózhó náhásdlíí' (May beauty be restored).
Hózhó náhásdlíí' (May beauty be restored).

Action/Reflection:

Talk to someone today about who/what you have lost in the pandemic.

Who and what have you lost in the pandemic? Reflect on this and write about it.

The Oxygen Cycle

With your permission, I would like to take us back to a scary place:6th grade science class: Braces. Awkwardness. Cooties. Scratchy voice. Hair growing in places it never grew before.

Sorry, if that makes you squirm. For 6th graders who are reading this, those are all compliments of your pre-teen development that adults "miss" dearly.

Now, call to mind your 6th grade science teacher and you might remember them introducing the Oxygen Cycle. Oxygen (O_2) is generated as a waste product of photosynthesis. This O_2 is given off by plants and then taken into the lungs of animals/ humans to sustain their lives. Animals/humans give off carbon dioxide (CO_2) as a waste product and that is soaked up by plants.

Now that I have you really smiling a big, pre-teen, mouth-of-braces, grin, I will share what this cycle really has to teach us. Oxygen. For us, it represents everything that sustains and supports us in this life. Call to mind the oxygen in your life – the people, the communities, the Higher Power, etc. that sustain you.

Oxygen Cycle on Earth

Take a few deep breaths and take in that oxygen that sustains life – literally and figuratively. Physically and metaphysically. Spiritually and in 6th grade form, pairs of oxygen atoms connected by a double bond.

Give thanks for the oxygen in your life.

But life cannot exist simply by breathing in. We must also exhale what is not needed. For us, that is CO_2, carbon dioxide.

Call to mind the carbon dioxide in your life – the elements of life that do not serve you being the best you. Things that hold you back. We all carry this CO_2 – fear, self-doubt, selfishness, trauma – as it is part of life, part of the Oxygen Cycle.

Give thanks for the carbon dioxide in your life.

Yes, as important as it is to give thanks and breathe in the O_2 of our lives, we can work toward a place of gratitude toward CO_2. We can also work on the practice of long, slow exhales and ways to release our CO_2.

There is nothing inherently wrong with the carbon dioxide in our lives as long as we have ways to release it. If left to build up in the body, CO_2 causes a medical condition known as hypercapnia which can be fatal. (For those that are curious, COVID-19 does cause respiratory failure but not elevated CO_2…but this blog is not about the pandemic, if you have been paying attention.)

Practice today, in the name of 6th grade science class and the Oxygen Cycle.

Deep breaths in – soak in that oxygen.

Deep breaths out - let go of your carbon dioxide.

Practice a loving mindset and heartset with both actions.

One last thought. It is profound to me that the same CO_2 waste product we expel is a life-giving force to the plants around us. Staring at my photosynthesizing relatives, I wonder if they have this same reflection as they watch us gobble up the O2 waste product they were all too eager to release.

Life is beautiful in that way. Not only do we participate in the Oxygen Cycle, but we do so inter-connected to each other in a way that sustains life for us all.

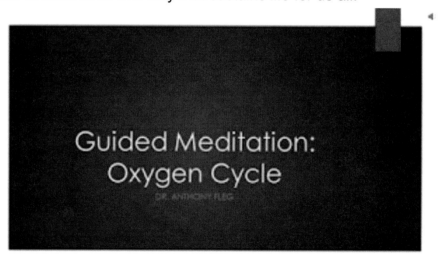

As an added bonus to this week's piece, I have recorded an 8-minute guided meditation using the Oxygen Cycle as our guide (geez, my 6th grade science teacher must be proud right now! Or ashamed. Either way, here it is: https://youtu.be/q27YEwPaQk8

Action/Reflection:
Write about your own perspective and insights on the oxygen cycle as it pertains to your life.

May 6, 2020

Corona – Tha Verse

This week's piece is a visual art/poetry collaboration. I gave the initial lines of this poem to collaborator Christian Gering, who worked on art that he felt embodied the poetry. See more of his art @ www.christiangering.com

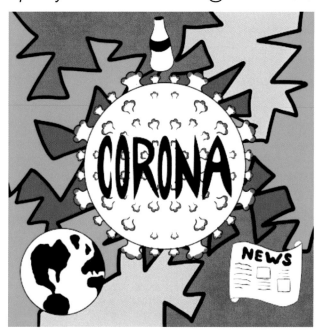

Corona

    beer or virus

    killers of livers

           lungs

              longevity

                life purpose

Corona

    "crown" en español

    symbol of colonizer's destiny manifested

            globe infected

            pandemic ignored

    not-so-covid operation

    dissecting

commodifying

all that is within

        and

    on

        Mother's Earth

unlike surgeon's scalpel

this infectious quest claiming no intention to heal

Corona

    La Rona

    SARS-CoV-2

        miniscule RNA sequence bringing down double-stranded DNA world

    (distinct from Ebola, H1N1 and others who have tried)

    has huddled humanity

stopped a world of speed

stripped us of the

        "social"

          into just

            "being"

Corona

    COVID

    "Mr. 19"

    Plague '20

        lurking in the shadows

        longing for host

        looking

          4

            way

              in

                2

                  lungs

Bringing

   us

    2

     our

      knees

       tears

       suffering

       pain

Bringing

   us

    2

     our

      knees

       prayerful

       grateful

       humbled

Corona,

 brothers and sisters is our 3-day Hogan healing,
 and we sit collectively in its first night

 This is Ceremony

    This is Beautyway*

 This is Enemyway*

 This is Hozho*

    This is Cleansing

    This is Renewal

    This is Healing

*Beautyway and Enemyway are names for traditional Navajo Ceremonies. Hozho is a Navajo concept invoking "peace, balance, harmony."

The Shoe-Less Hike

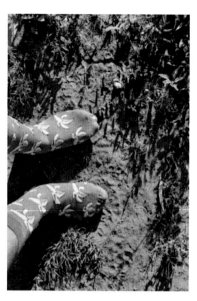

We had escaped to hike, a Mother's Day celebration.

I was depleted, finishing a 7-day stretch of hospital medicine in the new world order – face masks, globs of hand sanitizer, lonely patients, and some conversations reduced from in-person to tablets.

So depleted, in fact, that I worried if I could muster energy to make Mother's Day special for my wife.

"Get the kids ready, pack them in the car," I texted as I left the hospital.

I knew if I could avoid slumping into a chair or onto a bed, I had a chance.

So it went – "Dad's home" followed a minute later by the car starting our escape into the Sandia Mountains that shadow our city of Albuquerque.

We arrived. The ritual of checklist that comes with having four children began. Water bottles? Check. Sunscreen? Check. Hats? Check. All children present? Check.

All looked to be in order until my personal check. Shoes? Shoes? In my haste to leave, I had left shoes behind.Leaving me with a quick decision to make. Option 1: Smile and enjoy a shoe-less hike, saving our Mother's Day adventure from crashing to a halt. Option 2: "Everyone back in the car. Wave to the hike that would have been."
Option 1 is our world.

Making the best out of the less-than-optimal, far-from-normal options. Option 1 is virtual birthday parties, graduations, and weddings. Option 1 is our decision not to give up, not to give in, but to get creative.

So we hiked. Passerbys trying not to stare too long at my socks. A few made jokes. One family with young children asked "What happened to your shoes?" as they headed up the trail as we made our way back to the car.

"A bear just jumped out of nowhere and snatched them. Said he wanted Nikes."
The "really??" look on the faces was a small victory for my defeated feet, stinging from the rocks and roots incessantly poking from underneath. My wife, citing social decency

and Navajo tradition that says by naming an animal you call them to you, gave me *that look* ending my shoe-less victory dance.

My feet survived, the hike was saved, and Mother's Day happened. Maybe my feet were even strengthened by the uncomfortable experience.

Today will give us such moments, with an Option 1 in each case that does not feel like the right answer, but which is the best option.

Pick Option 1. Be proud. Get excited for what this path might hold. Feel free to laugh - at yourself, at your feet, at the moment - if needed.

Option 1, as a friend reminded is simply this: "Don't fight the current, find the current and flow with it."

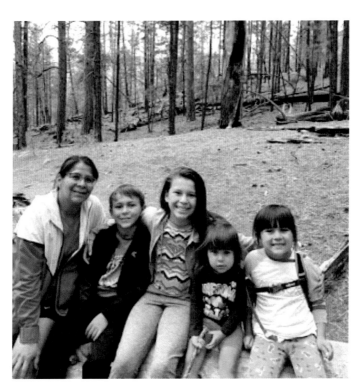

My 5 biggest motivations to go with Option 1 (from L-R are my wife Shannon, son Bah'hozhooni, and daughters Nizhoni, Sihasin and Shandiin)

Action/Reflection:

Take special care to notice today when you have to choose something that is not the ideal, an Option 1.

Write about a time recently where you chose Option 1.

When Life Gives You Lemons...Fermentation Begins

Chef Joe Romero (Navajo/Hopi/Zuni/Taos) and I connected over food, healthy and creative food to be exact. He has offered his time and talents to NHI's "Food is Medicine" 6-week challenges, with recipes that "remix" the ideas around sustainability, affordability and "make-ability" (e.g.) someone without the title 'chef' can actually produce it).

Some of his creations were so packed with life and art and creative energy that I started writing spoken word poetry inspired by his recipes. Well, this will give you a taste of the creative energy.
– in this case, he took a piece from this blog and created a recipe he felt expressed the piece in a culinary form. I then took his savory lemon recipe and wrote a short piece of poetry to add even more flavor – this follows his recipe below. Get your tastebuds ready!

FROM CHEF JOE

Inspired by the words of Dr. Fleg and his kids' response to these uncertain times, I too was trying to see the light in this situation.

After reading the blog "A Gratitude Perspective On Coronavirus", I asked myself, "How can one turn some invisible microbes and bacteria into a blessing?" Then it hit me like a rotting tomato-fermentation!

So many of our everyday and favorite foods are fermented blessings - coffee, chocolate, bread, and hot sauces to name a few.

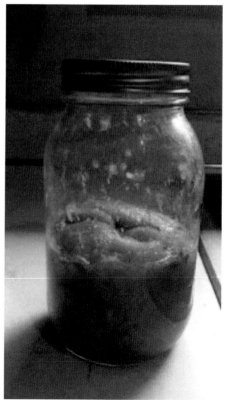

In the fermenting process we harness the microbes in the air to interact and create beneficial bacteria in simple ingredients to transform and aid flavor development and to preserve.

Bonus! These foods boost our immune system too!

Rotting food – noxious or nourishing? It is all in how you choose to digest it!

So with no further delay, here is a recipe for one of my favorite kitchen blessings, culinary art inspired by the first piece of this blog adventure.

Find the recipe on the following page!

PRESERVED LEMONS

When life gives you lemons…you ferment those beauties!
The bright citrus flavor of fermented lemons, balanced by brininess and sourness, can add so much depth and nuance to so many dishes. Try adding to your salsas, pan sauces, and yogurt toppings for both savory and sweet applications. This can be added anywhere you would add regular lemon – have fun experimenting!

Ingredients:

12 Lemons (4 scrubbed and dried, 8 juiced to yield 1 1/2 cups), plus extra juice if needed
1/2 cup Kosher Salt.

Recipe:

Cut lemons lengthwise into quarters, stopping 1 inch from bottom so lemons stay intact at base.

Hold 1 lemon over medium bowl and pour 2 tablespoons salt into its cavity. Gently rub cut surfaces of lemon together, then place in clean 1 quart jar. Repeat with remaining lemons and salt. Add any accumulated salt and juice in bowl to jar.

Pour 1 1/2 cups lemon juice into jar and press gently to submerge lemons. Add more lemon juice to jar needed to cover lemons completely. Cover jar tightly with lid and shake.

Refrigerate lemons, shaking jar once per day for first 4 days to redistribute salt and juice. Let lemons cure in refrigerator until glossy and softened, usually 6 to 8 weeks. (Preserved lemons can be refrigerated for up to 6 months.)

Cut off desired amount of preserved lemon. Using knife, remove pulp and white pith from rind.
Slice, chop, or mince rind as desired. Only the rind is usable.

"Lemon madness
Digging
Deep
Into tastebuds treasury
Waste product no more
Lacto-fermentation, wearing Superwoman's cape,
Has saved the day
Has reminded us of the cycle of life
Has begged us not give up when things begin to spoil, soil, rot, ferment.
Has begged us to have faith and simply stay (in)tuned –
This is where new life, new taste
Blossoms
Blooms
Explodes
Expands

Mind and mouth consciousness of
what was
and what is
and
what *can be*"

Flow With It

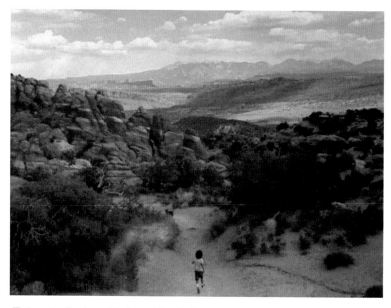

About this picture: Taken in Arches National Park (Utah), it reminds us in a very real way of the healing power of movement. There is a saying "dogs and kids are happiest when running"; here you will see our 3 year-old son Bah'Hozhooni running after our dog. My corollary to this saying is that our goal as adults is to keep the child within alive. Movement = Medicine.

Slow. Sluggish. Feet dragging. Legs heavy.

The run was not the effortless morning wake-up I had envisioned when I sat on front steps tying the shoes. The gazelle I had envisioned, gently bouncing over the trails, had turned into more of a hippo waddling along.

Then, around 15 minutes into the run, I remembered a friend's wisdom. "Don't fight the current. Find it and flow with it."

So, flow with it became my mantra.

As a competitive runner, flowing at an admittedly pedestrian speed is sort of new. But then again, I am a competitive runner 3 months into a pandemic, exhausted from work as a family physician to support others in movement and health. I am a runner whose competition has become measured by resilience more than by mile pace or race times/awards.

It took some effort, but over the next miles of the run I repeated flow with it and let the run take over. Suddenly, the trees seemed more present. The flowering plants of our New

Before I realized it, I was in that wonderful space that running offers us, escape from pandemic and all of life's stressors. I hardly noticed that my pace had quickened.

Flow with it.

hat's my prescription for us all. Let your movement be medicine on all levels – mind, body and spirit. Let your runs/walks/hikes/dance/gardening/etc. be a way to connect with yourself and nature in a way that we know is deep in our DNA as humans: running. As we see a world suffering, dedicate your movement to the healing of those infected and all of us affected.

Flow with it.

And in the fine print of the prescription, I might also add that flow with it means to take care of being gentle with ourselves in this moment. Your movement is a chance to make space for yourself, but make sure that space is healing, loving, uplifting. Flow with it and appreciate your body for what it is doing, not what it isn't doing.

On some pandemic days, gentleness with ourselves is going to mean throwing out the pace or mileage goal for the day; instead, focusing on being present, giving thanks for the moment and gratitude for your body that allows you the gift of that day's movement.

As we say in our Running Medicine program, "Breathe deep, forget all worries, and get your medicine.

May your movement be wonderful and healing today. May you have the strength and presence to...

Flow with it.

Action/Reflection:

Flow with it today, especially in the moments that feel the hardest to do so.

Write about a moment recently where you chose to flow with it.

White Supremacy: Time to Cure the Disease

White supremacy.

I look at those two words and breathe deep.

Can I find healing in those words and what they represent?

Here goes.

Two initial thoughts to help frame this conversation.

As a physician, I know the importance of distinguishing diseases from symptoms. For example, pneumonia is the disease that causes symptoms of cough, fever, and shortness of breath. We know in medicine that **treating the downstream symptoms without addressing the disease causing those symptoms is not effective**. We don't treat the cough, we treat the pneumonia causing the cough.

White supremacy is the disease, racism is the symptom of the disease.

Second, a concept from systems theory: **Every system is perfectly designed to get the results it gets**. This reminds us that moments like this week are not about who is "racist" and who is not. It isn't about the police officers that brutally murdered George Floyd (RIP) or the deranged duo that attacked and killed Ahmaud Arbery (RIP). It is about the system that is perfectly designed for events like these to happen over and over in a systemic way.

Back to white supremacy.

White supremacy is the disease we still do not talk about. Especially as white people.

Racism is a symptom of this disease. It pervades our societies and globe where white supremacy thrives.

Allow me to define white supremacy. It is not goons in white hooded robes burning crosses and terrorizing communities of color as most of us have been led to believe, a convenient way of letting the rest of us white folks off the hook. **White supremacy is the belief that white people are superior to those of all other races and should therefore dominate society**. It is behind such concepts as *manifest destiny* and the genocide inflicted on brown and black populations of the globe as white Europeans decided in some pseudo-religious hallucination that the world was theirs for the taking.

They didn't need to state as they pillaged and raped people and their lands that this quest was "in the name of white supremacy." Look at the results, so clearly divided along the lines of skin color and it becomes crystal clear that the system here is white supremacy, perfectly designed to get the results it gets.

White supremacy, through its symptom of racism, leads blacks being killed by police at a rate three times that of whites. It is why the shootings of black men and cases of missing and murdered Indigenous women, in a repeated and predictable way, seem less important to investigate.

In this pandemic, white supremacy is behind communities of color bearing the biggest burden of death during COVID. American Indians make up 11% of New Mexico but account for an astounding 57% of our COVID cases. When we look at factors leading to this high rate, white people seem suddenly appalled to learn about sub-standard housing and rampant poverty and unemployment in our Indigenous Nations. They feign shock and dismay at hearing that 30% of houses on the Navajo Nation lack running water.

White supremacy places these communities, these brown lives as less important. As a white person, I am responsible for these conditions that lead to a very predictable outcome when a pandemic or other natural disaster hits.

Look at our prisons, look at our communities with the worst schools and least job prospects, look at our communities who live sickest and die youngest, look at places where the toxic waste dumps are put. We all know too well the color of those populations and it ain't white.

As a white person, I must own my complicity in this being our current reality.

My healing begins here, in owning white supremacy as something that has gotten me into doors and places I didn't deserve and as something I inflict through my whiteness and through my actions on people of color around me. As a person whose whiteness has given me un-earned privilege each day of my life, this moment gives me and people like me a chance to truly work for a cure to white supremacy. Forget support groups and self-help books about how to be less racist – I want to be a part in curing the white supremacy disease that causes racism.

I challenge my white colleagues to join me in having tough conversations with ourselves and our inner circle of family and friends. Robin DiAngelo, a scholar who coined a term *white fragility* proposes that whites are "socialized into a deeply internalized sense of superiority and entitlement that we are either not consciously aware of or can never admit to ourselves, we become highly fragile in conversations about race." Let's break out of that paralyzing place and start thinking and talking about white supremacy.

But that improved insight will change exactly nothing. Turning that into actions that overturn white supremacy in our workplaces, in our neighborhoods, in our systems. This needs to be our commitment. No more asking people of color to cure the disease that whites created and need to fix.

White supremacy.

I am still trying to get comfortable with saying it and acknowledging my part in its devilish, racist plot.

But if we, white people, begin there, it is a great start.

If we start to understand, we can begin to act.

And in understanding and acting, that is where, my brothers and sisters, healing begins.

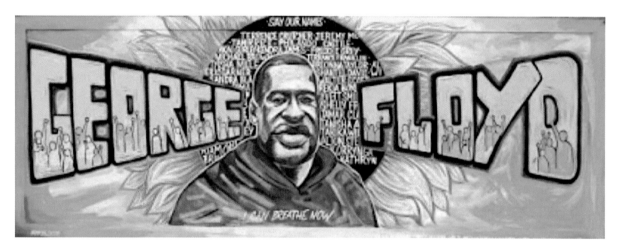

Note: I want to credit and thank one of my mentors in all things social justice, Tonya Covington, who gave me needed insight on white supremacy that led to this piece. Thank you Tonya!

Action Challenge:
Has White Supremacy unfairly aided you or hindered you in your life? Have a courageous conversation this week about this.

If you identify as a White, choose a small step you can take in "curing the disease" of White Supremacy. For example, reading more on the subject, talking about this openly with co-workers or family, etc.

Strawberry Wisdom

"I just want a few berries."

This was my comment that started the earthy discussion. We were visiting with friends who have a thriving garden producing more than they can consume.

As we talked about the types of lettuce and greens in the neatly organized rows, I heard mention of strawberries.

No offense to the other things growing, but the mention of berries had me dialed in. Where? How many? Ready to pick?

We walked over to the berry bushes, new plantings this year and I got news that made my stomach groan. Literally.

"The berries won't be here until next year. See, if you want a strawberry bush to put its energy into growing deep, strong roots you actually clip the flowers as they arise in the first year. You don't want it putting energy toward producing flowers and berries. You want it to put its energy toward growing strong roots for lots of berries in the years to come."

Many reading this will question why they are even reading this series, an author who doesn't have a grasp of the simplest of growing concepts. An author whose quest for berries clouds his view of the bigger picture. Understood. Exit doors at the rear.

But, for those still reading, I ask us what these strawberry plants have to teach us in the bigger picture as we grapple with our twin pandemics of COVID and white supremacy.

Yes, we all want berries. Right now.

We want to find a fix to the pesky Coronavirus reality that doesn't quite have any quick, easy, right-answer angles. Open up society!!!! 😐😐😐 Open up society???? 😟😟😟 Open up society!!!!???? 😖😖😖 Not sure what punctuation or emoji to give it, and I sense that most of us feel this way. And the deeper questioning from the pandemic - how do we want to be as communities and as a society once it has passed?

We want to immediately produce berries to begin fixing a white supremacy problem that has grown deep roots over 500 plus years.

Maybe it is a moment not for berries, but for preparing for berries that will come in the future. That's right taste buds, just hold tight.

And the strawberry plants remind us that sometimes life gives us a tough either/or decision. A decision my friend and I discussed right there in the garden, out of earshot from the strawberry bushes themselves. "Don't you think we could just trick them into a few flowers, a few berries this year??" I whispered.

By focusing on the immediate moment ("Berries! Now!"), succumbing to our desire to taste that unique seed-laden sweetness that leaks its scarlet juice as we munch, we sabotage the bigger picture for growth, for fruit in the future. We sabotage our own intentions and efforts toward change.

In writing today, I thought of two pieces of wisdom from some of the wonderful "gardners" in my life..

One mentor reminded, "The breath in stillness also invigorates."

A mentee said it this way: "The pandemic and everything going on in our society is definitely exhausting but I find it a little easier when I focus on what I can do now as my own person and my own biases. Working on that is what will start change."

These two pandemics of our current moment implore us to put energy into growing roots for healing and reconciliation with our planet, with ourselves, and with each other.

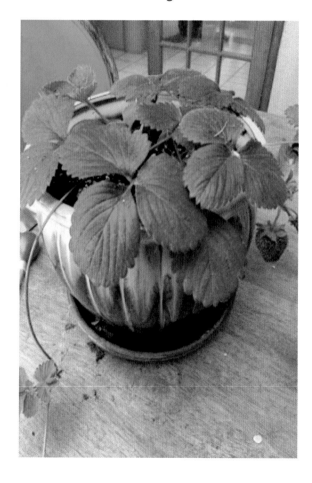

While a few berries might feed us in the present, the best gardening we can do now is to work for berries that will nourish in the years and generations to come.

Action/Reflection:

In what way has the pandemic helped you to focus on growing strong roots as opposed to working for a few berries in the moment? Write a reflection piece on this.

Photo: A young strawberry plant, just added to our family. Initially, we wanted berries this year. Now, our attention and energy is to guide it to dig strong, deep roots. A few berries bear witness to our prior mindset :)

"There is Still Normal" vs. "Nothing is Normal"

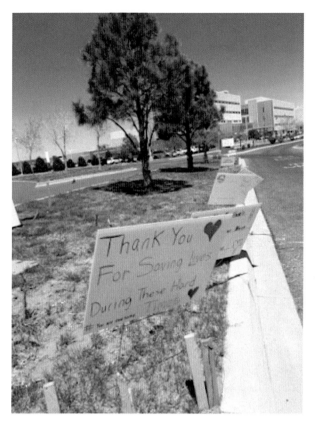

Signs. Bagpipes. Cursing.

I approach the hospital, a real live doctor in a virtual world here to provide real live healing.

Like all of us, I vacillate between "There is still normal" and "Nothing is normal" each pandemic day. Arriving at the hospital, stethoscope gently embracing my neck, I try to convince myself of the former.

These three reminders shove me toward the latter.

Signs. Bagpipes. Cursing.

The line of signs make me gasp, all along entrance into the hospital. Some printed and professional. But the ones that induce tear ducts into action are the handmade ones.

"For the time you spend helping me when I am sick, Thank You."

"Whether it is a headache, fever or the flu, no illness stands a chance against a doctor like you!"

"Thank you for saving lives during these hard times. # You are awesome."

I walk over to have a moment with the row of signs. Gratitude for this display of kindness we are seeing in the last months. Not just for health care workers. But gratitude for all who keep on putting themselves at risk to keep food on our table, all who keep our cities and towns safe and functional. Gratitude toward the parents-turned-school teachers and for the teachers and barbers and shopkeepers and neighbors, everyone who brings joy and meaning to our lives.

The signs - a signal of the wave of kindness this collective moment has inspired.

Bagpipes.

As I stand with the signs, I am not sure I am hearing right. Being a family physician, I immediately think of the most likely diagnosis: auditory hallucination. But the music continues. Approaching the hospital entrance, the bagpipe player comes into view.

Living in New Mexico, these Scottish instruments do not often grace our presence. Definitely not in hospital entranceways. I listen to the slow, mournful wailing.

The bagpipes speak very clearly to me as I watch a group of health care workers take in the melody. It is a moment to heal together, people needing strength to go back inside and care for those weakened by disease. Yes, we did have a few hospitalized with COVID, but the bigger population needing us are the non-COVID patients who lay socially isolated in scary hospital rooms, stripped of family members at bedside due to the pandemic.

The bagpipes a signal of the collective suffering to be acknowledged and the ways we find meaning in coming together to mourn, grieve, cry, and wail.

But I wasn't in the building yet. A loud argument reaches my ears. Two cars, drivers shouting at top of lungs to each other. Seemingly, one had stripped the varnish off the other's humanity by some move on the highway. (We call this "New Mexico Drivers Syndrome). Do they not realize all of us can hear them. Do they not see the signs or hear the bagpipes in front of them?

I guess in a way this is a nice complement to the other two. A showing of raw emotion, escalated by the pandemic pressure cooker in which we all find ourselves huddled.

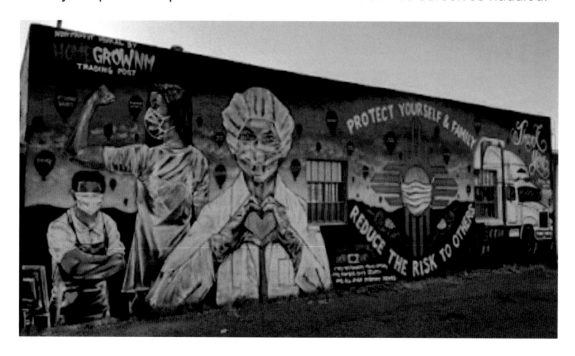

Let it out. Curse it out. "This cursing could even be healthy healing in a virtual world without outlets for stress relief,"the Socrates in me ponders.

Now, I am really stuck.

I have yet to even step foot in the building to hear what has changed since a week earlier.

I have not even gotten to the part where I learn how my social etiquette for today includes things I never thought to do (or not do) just days prior.

I have yet to even step foot in the building to hear what has changed since a week earlier. I have not even gotten to the part where I learn how my social etiquette for today includes things I never thought to do (or not do) just days prior.

I can't even get there because I am stuck on signs of kindness, pipes of mourning, and stress-induced cursing. All three the raw emotions of the moment. Nothing needing to be processed or diagnosed. But simply gulped down along with the fresh New Mexico air of the day as something true to the moment.

Gathering myself, I step toward the front door, one thing cleared up for the moment debate between "There is still normal" and "Nothing is normal" is quite clear.

Action/Reflection:

Go out of your way this week to thank someone for the work they do. Mail carrier,cashier at grocery store, etc. Watch how good it feels – for you and them!

Love for Community - the Emelia Pino Story

She saw a community hurting, struggling.

She is from Zia Pueblo, sitting northwest of the Albuquerque/Rio Rancho area. Zia was one of the first Indigenous communities to be hard-hit by COVID cases and deaths in a state where an alarming majority of COVID cases are among Native Americans.

She, is Emelia Pino, daughter of Charlotte and Fernando Pino.

Emelia is one of 6 children, with four older sisters and a younger brother. She is a senior at Bernalillo High School who plans to become a pediatrician, and someone I got to meet over this last year as she was a part of Native Health Initiative's Healers of Tomorrow (HOT) program.

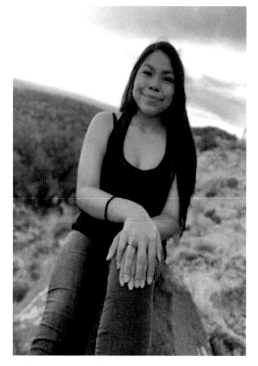

Make no mistake: Emelia is a healer of today. She saw a shortage of PPE in her community and set out to fix it. She saw a shortage of PPE in her community and set out to fix it.

"Our community is hurting. We have lost a few of our elders. Being that we are such a close-knit community, it really hurt me to see my community struggling. I don't see youth taking a lead in my community but I felt it was time to stand up and make a difference."

1,400 masks and a variety of sanitation supplies resulted from her standing up. But she was not done. She saw youth hurting in a different way, isolated under Zia's strict orders that those under 18 are not allowed to leave the Pueblo. The mandate is intended to keep these youth and the Zia Pueblo community safe. But, Emelia saw the way it has affected her peers, especially now that the school year is over.

So, Emelia Pino, healer of today, went to work. She wanted all 270 youth to receive an educational kit with age-appropriate books, games, and supplies. She wrote a grant, something that most folks twice her age shudder to think about doing.

So, Emelia Pino, healer of today, went to work. She wanted all 270 youth to receive an educational kit with age-appropriate books, games, and supplies. She wrote a grant, something that most folks twice her age shudder to think about doing.

As I write this, she is collecting donations of money and supplies and working to bring joy with these care packages over the next weeks. Not stressing about how it is all going to happen, or about the summer break ticking away. In fact, she is already thinking about how to inspire other youth to step up and lead similar efforts in their Tribes and communities. **Love for community** – that is something we maybe have overlooked during the pandemic. It is something that Emelia reminds us a true way to actualize a gratitude perspective on Coronavirus.

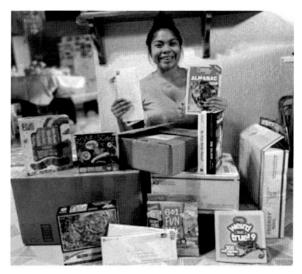

Step up, stand up, and make things happen. Emelia, I am now writing to you personally. Thank you. Thank you for showing us that all of us can be great, as all of us can serve. Thank you for reminding us of the creativity and leadership that youth have for changing our world, not tomorrow, but today, right now.

Thank you. Thank you for showing us that all of us can be great, as all of us can serve. Thank you for reminding us of the creativity and leadership that youth have for changing our world, not tomorrow, but today, right now. Thank you for loving your community, Zia Pueblo, in a way that inspires me and all of us to greater service and action. (*Emelia, if you blush reading this, that's cool. No one is watching. They promised not to look*).

Note: when this blog was originally posted, we invited people to support Emelia's donation drive.

Action/Reflection:

Go out of your way to give a gift to someone this week. Maybe a letter sharing your appreciation for a co-worker. A gift card for a stranger. Give from the heart and see what happens

Celebrating Inter-Dependence this July 4th!

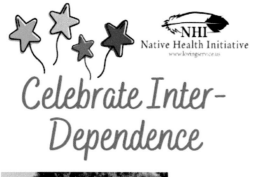

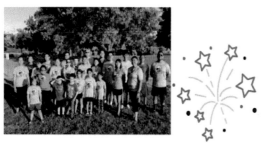

Having turned the corner into the second half of 2020, July 4th upon us, we have a unique moment in which to consider celebrating "independence" or "inter-dependence".

Inter-dependence has nothing to do with patriotism. It is about who we are as humans and our profound connection to each other, to all living things, to the air and land and water.

The pandemic has gently guided us to seeing how interconnected we are, while the mass demonstrations are a plea for recognizing and valuing each beautiful human being, a foundation to showing our inter-dependence upon one another.

I think of a hike I took not long ago with my brother Jerome in northern California. Sugarloaf State Park, to be exact. The area had been hit with devastating wildfires in 2018 and the forest showed its scars – burnt trees lined much of the hike. But as I scanned my vision upward, I saw something unexpected. I blinked to make sure I was not imagining it.

Out of a blackened tree trunk vibrant green sprigs of leaves grew at the top.

And this was not limited to one "miracle tree". This was strongly a theme, a pattern to the forest one year after the fires. Add in the moss and other growths beginning to inhabit the burnt trunk and it became suddenly clear this scene was much more complex than a deadened forest. New life, resilience now the title of the portrait.

Yes, even life and death show inter-dependence on one another, speaks the forest. The courageous audacity of life to think that it can spring up from a tree burned to a crisp is amazing, beautiful, inspiring. Within our lives, we can call to mind places of hurt, sorrow, trauma that then grew from that very branch a new leaf.

My friends, inter-dependence, once realized, changes how we treat those around us and the planet we inhabit. It changes how we see suffering in our fellow humans and in our natural world. May this year's fireworks spark a celebration of inter-dependence in all of us.

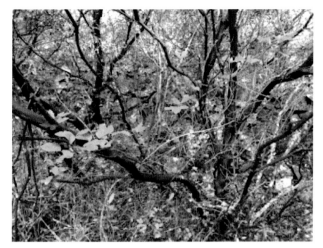

Life and death dance around each other in the wake of forest fires Sugarloaf State Park, California

Two additional items:

* What is 4th of July without some amazing food? Chef Joe Romero, my dear friend and creative collaborator, thought about a recipe that spoke about inter-dependence to him, and came up with Red Chile Vinaigrette (recipe below). In his words:

Nature is abundant, it is diverse, and it has more varieties than we can guess. We need to grow and eat a diverse diet full of different colors, textures, shapes, and sizes.

We also need to cultivate meaningful relationships with the diverse people that grow our food and the people that transform that food into love and culture, thus ensuring healthy bodies, healthy soil and a healthy mind.

When I need my large dose of local organic produce I turn to a big salad. Nothing is so effortlessly beautiful and delicious as a bowl of mixed greens and chopped colorful fresh veggies. Next, the dressing to bring it all together; Red Chile Vinaigrette. I have not found a salad that this spicy sweet vinaigrette does not compliment well. Make sure to share with friends and family and total strangers.

* Buddhist teacher and activist Thich Nhat Hanh (Rest in Peace) talks about "inter-being". I learned a good amount about this amazing teacher who was nominated for the Nobel Peace Prize by Dr. Martin Luther King in writing tonight's piece.

I found his 14 guidelines for Inter-Being to be quite grounding in thinking about how inter-dependence relates to my own actions regarding racial and planet justice.

Given that no one was up at the 1am hour to grant me permission to re-publish those 14 guidelines, I have a link here to a 1995 interview of him that includes the guidelines.

THREE SISTERS KITCHEN
NOURISHING EACH OTHER FROM THE GROUND UP

Salad with Red Chile Vinaigrette
by chef Joe Romero
serves 4-6

Ingredients:

½ cup rice vinegar
1/3 cup water
½ Tablespoon black pepper
1 Tablespoon salt
3 Tablespoons honey, or to taste
3 Tablespoons red chile powder
½ cup olive oil
your favorite salad greens (lettuce, spinach, arugula etc.)
a handful of pecans, toasted and chopped

Instructions:

1. Add rice vinegar, water, black pepper, salt, honey, and red chile powder to a blender or a small bowl.

2. *If using a blender:* turn the speed up slowly and add the olive oil in a slow steady stream until your dressing is well blended.
If using a bowl: whisk the dressing in a small bowl, while adding the olive oil in a slow steady stream. Whisk until well blended.

3. Taste to make sure you like the seasoning – add more chile, black pepper, or salt to taste, if needed.

4. Toss salad greens with toasted pecans and drizzle with vinaigrette, a tablespoon at a time, until the leaves are lightly coated with dressing.

I Am Sorry

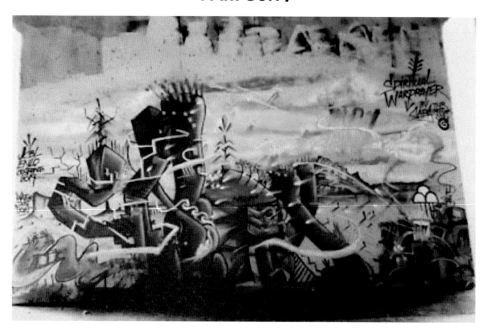

Spiritual Warprayer by Saba (2019)

This week's piece is an apology. Like everything else I have written over the past 4 months, it is from the heart. That is the only place from which I know to write.

As we hear society suddenly "awakened" to the racism of mascots, statues, and even the food pantry's pancake syrup and processed food rice, I hear a sentiment that goes something like this. "We have now come to realize that this image, this stereotype, this caricature of a group of people is racist."

I don't buy it, and it isn't about pointing the finger at anyone.

I am certain that like me, all of white America has known and always understood that these images were about dehumanizing our communities of color. We just chose to do nothing.

Now, where it is socially safe and financially beneficial to act are we making change happen.

But let's be real.

Let's be honest.

Let's be humble and sincere.

We knew all along that these images were part of a sick plot to dehumanize our beautiful brothers and sisters of color.

Change is good to see, but white folks like myself and institutions that are changing would do well to add an apology.

For healing on all levels, "I am sorry" matters.
~~~~~~~~~~~~~~~~~~~~~~~~~~~~~~~~~~~~~~~

Don Juan de Onate.

I remember when I moved to New Mexico, hearing the history of Onate from Acoma Pueblo and then trying to figure out why he and so many symbols of genocide are revered hundreds of years later in a land that claims to respect and value diversity. I saw that there was an Onate Hall on our UNM campus and had a hard time understanding how orchestrating a campaign of murder and torture on Acoma Pueblo earns you the right to have a building named after you. Or why one of the city's nicest parks, tucked in along the Bosque was named Kit Carson after another murderer whose "scorched earth" campaign says all you need to know about his legacy.

As a white person, I didn't appreciate the violence that statues and other signs of reverence perpetuate on people and communities of color. I chose to do nothing.

Imagine an Indigenous youngster with family outside of the ABQ Museum asking mom and dad why this person who tortured their ancestors is given a heroic statue. Or being a first generation college student of color at UNM and attending your ethnic studies class in Onate Hall.

I am sorry.

I also failed to realize what it says about our society that continues to accept this reality. Here is exactly what it says:

1) We value conquistadors and the legacy of violent, brutal conquest more than we value the original inhabitants of this land.

2) It says loud and clear that we continue to tell a story of whose land this is and how it was obtained in a way that psychiatrists would label delusional (e.g. not based in reality).

3) It says that white supremacy, a belief that white people are superior to those of all other races and should therefore dominate society, is alive and well, not limited to extremists and hate groups.

4) It says that we think it is okay to keep people of color in a perpetual state of fear as a means of exerting power and control over them.

5) It reminds me that white privilege blinds me from a large part of reality in this country (e.g. everyone's reality who is not white) and that I need to listen deeply to what communities of color are saying if I want to have any bit of those blinders removed.

I am proud of my city, Albuquerque, that is on its way to removing all remnants of this delusional way of being from our midst. I don't just want to see the statues and names removed – I want to apologize deeply for my inaction that kept these changes from happening sooner. I chose to do nothing, despite the moral compass that told me that Onate and Carson types have no place in the 21st century.

I am complicit in this violence of inaction.

I am ready to change our landscape, starting with my own mind and heart that tells me whether or not to stand up and act when I see others dehumanized.

I am sorry.

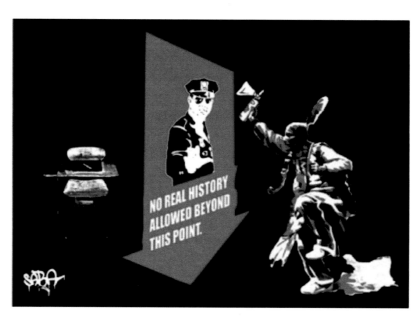

*Randy Sabaque (Jemez Pueblo/Dine'), known in the art/hip hop world as "Saba",
has always inspired me to see deeper through his art. I am honored to include
these two pieces of his as part of this week's blog. The first piece
"Spiritual Warprayer" in Saba's words, "shows little villages at the bottom
fighting massive skyscraping structures sucking from the earth, from those villages.
The rain and ancestors are working to cleanse the destruction.*

Action/Reflection:
If you were to write a letter similar to this piece, titled "I am sorry" who would you write it to? Write the piece and deliver it. You could also deliver this verbally, as opposed to writing it.

Kindness (aka Love for Community Part 2: The Nehemiah Cionelo Story)

Kindness.

Have you noticed it around us these last months, often in bigger ways and larger doses than normal?

Think back to March/April when this was all starting. The acts of kindness that sprouted up like beautiful flowers that had been below the surface just waiting to break ground were right in our neighborhoods.

What random acts of kindness do you remember noticing in your neighborhood, in your life? Call those to mind right now. I promise, it will be good for you.

One day, at our mailbox, 4 ladybug rocks showed up. I still don't know the gifter and I looked down the street to see a young lady who had decorated her family's trashcans to

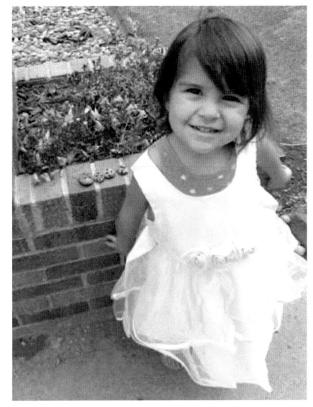

let the workers know how much they are appreciated.

I noticed the makeshift signs and art on the trails I run, people going out of their way to share their love. I paid attention to the neighbor's sign "Silence is violence" among the other signs affirming human dignity for all persons.

Kindness is one of the mechanisms for us healing in this moment, turning from politicized battles over mask-wearing, the latest depressing updates on the economy, and doomsday predictions to instead seeing the ways that our neighbors are being changed for the better by the pandemic. And if we pay attention to those ways that others are being changed, kindness becomes the change within.

In this blogosphere space, I had thought about how to elevate kindness, especially in seeing its absence in the stories and media I see in the pandemic.

Well, a few weeks ago I share the story of Emelia Pino and her service out of the love of her community of Zia Pueblo. Looking back, it was kindness finding its way into this blog before I realized what had happened.

And now, I am gifted with another kindness story to tell.

Hi Coach Fleg!

I hope you and your family are healthy and well right now.

I really would like to help out the community amidst what going on right now and I've been brainstorming how for a while. I understand food banks are under a lot of strain right now so I came up with the outlined fundraiser to help them out. Essentially, during a 12 hour period, I would try to run as many miles as I could. In turn, people would pledge to donate something like $25 for each of those miles. At the end of the day, the money raised would be able to go to some of Albuquerque's food banks.

This was how Nehemiah Cionelo (who goes by the name Nemo) pitched his idea to me in May, an idea to use his legs as a collegiate athlete for something much bigger than race awards. He had a name for the event, Footsteps for Families.

His motivation for this?

He shared that as a child in a big family where at times they barely got by, he could relate to what families like his must be dealing with in the pandemic.

"I wonder about if I were born 5 years later and were a teenager right now, what struggle I would be going through. Would I get any back to school supplies, for instance?" he commented.

The kindness in this case actually didn't completely surprise me. I have known this young man for close to a decade and he is one of those people who can achieve big things but never lose their humility and sense of belonging to a larger community.

Nemo's kindness has been a part of my daily life for the last weeks, and I am thankful for the 13-mile "running meeting" where we came up with the school supplies drive idea, text conversations, email and phone communication. Each and every one of them was kindness being poured into my life, me as the student listening to Nemo, my teacher.

Nemo with his siblings Moriah, Celeb, Gideon and Tabitha and Moriah's son Zyden

This Saturday I will proudly lace up the shoes to run some miles with him as we work to generate 1,000 miles over a 12 hour period, hoping to raise $10,000 for local families in need.

And I always believe that kindness is something to be shared and spread, so here is your chance to be involved in Footsteps for Families this Saturday, July 18th! (See below)

Notice kindness.

Generate kindness.

Spread it freely, my brothers and sisters.

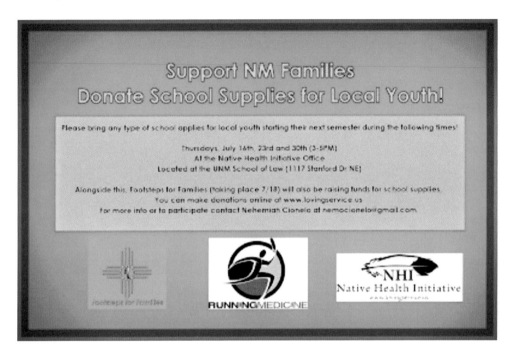

Action/Reflection:
Find a way to gift your community this week, following Nemo's example.

Renewal

Renewal
Even with 2020 vision
it often evades sight
blinded by our hurt and despair

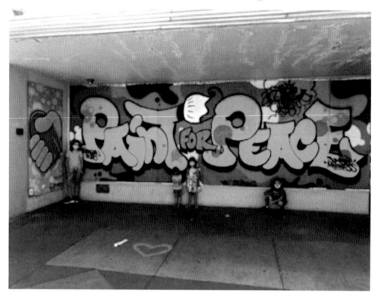

Renewal
is that precious flower that found crack in endless concrete
is that honey produced by our bee relatives from nectar source sour
is that child who "makes it out" in a system designed to keep her locked up, trapped in

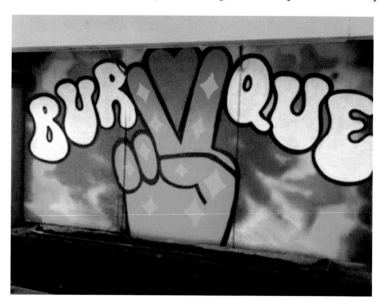

Renewal
hit me like a torrential monsoon rain
Creator's Tears
washing away
my fears
that downtown ABQ would stay in its
plywood plight
a reminder of an already struggling not-so-iconic Rte 66
mix
of
brothers and sisters discarded
businesses pandemiced
and cries for justice

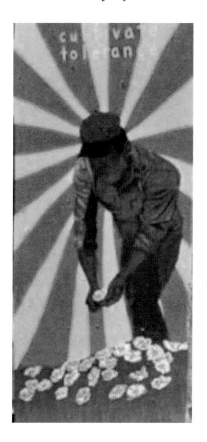

That was b4 the paint brushes, the Krylon
that smoothed over
plywood plight
doubt
fear
shame
wounds worn heavy like jeans in the rain

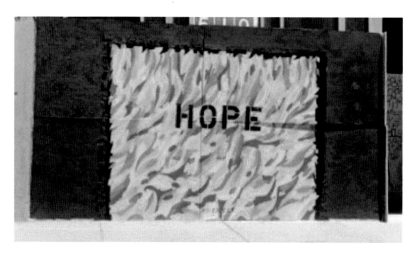

Paint for Peace, they call it
renewal through hope's tints, colors, hues,
brushing
dignity
pride
love
unity
back onto the canvas

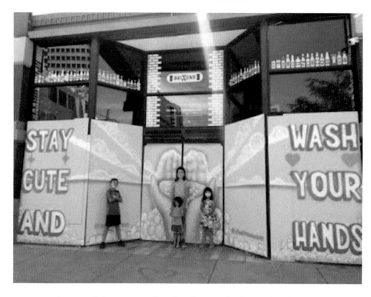

Author's note: There was plywood to cover the broken windows in downtown ABQ, an eyesore for an already struggling downtown. Well, a group of artists calling the project "Paint for Peace" decided to use that same plywood to beautify downtown with messages of hope, inspiration, love, unity. The pics shown here are part of this project. Go down and see it for yourself! TheAlibi did an article on Paint for Peace - https://alibi.com/art/60923/Paint-for-Peace-505.html.

Action/Reflection:

Find something you can do this week that will help you find renewal.

Of Tree Lines and Tolerance

We climbed and climbed. Endless "up" it seemed.

Finally, we got to a place with vistas endless. 360 degrees doesn't quite do it justice.

Christian, my running buddy and a professional trail runner, had brought me to Penitente Peak in the Santa Fe Mountains, 12,200 above sea level.

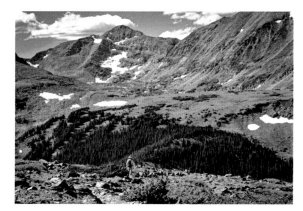

Our conversation over the first hours of the run had prepared us well for this peak. In fact, we talked about the Islamic tradition that talks about nature's beauty as the first tier of heaven.

Well, we had arrived in a place that inspired nothing short of otherworldly splendor.

Being an animal not used to such heights, I stared at the bare faces of the mountains at our eye level. Beneath that nakedness, pinons and spruce trees.

I had never climbed high enough to see what the "tree line" really was. I was now here.

I stared for a moment, confused a bit as I saw a clump of trees very much making a wavy line at best. Gone were my notions that the tree line would bring me back to high school geometry, a straight line connecting two points. Gone was my conceptualization of a belt that the mountain would wear around its waist, somewhere around 11,000 feet high.

I think Christian saw my look of surprise as I squinted to make sure I was seeing it all correctly.

"What was the tree line's teaching for me?" I thought as we began our descent.

My mind, and I assume most of ours, wants to see this world in a very straight-line way. Trees either grow or they don't, with a nice geometry-teacher-approved-line separating the two realities.

Tolerance requires us to see the trees for how they actually are, even if it jars us from a cemented belief not based in reality. Much more messy, akin to a 4 year old with a paintbrush in her hand as opposed to a ruler-drawn line.

Tolerance is a mindset that appreciates and looks for the nuances that make people who they are, seeking to understand their perspective, affirming their humanity and their right to think and behave differently.

It is a heartset that assumes commonality despite outward differences toward things we care about passionately like climate change, racism, or our best choice for president of the country. That commonality becomes the basis for tolerance, listening, and being open to change ourselves.

I did some reading on tree lines. Yes, they can be well-defined, but they are often a gradual transition. Trees grow shorter and more sparsely before gradually decreasing to an area with no trees. And depending on how the sun hits and where the water runs, the tree line likely differs in altitude even within a single mountain. There can even be a double tree line, with bristlecone pine trees growing far above the tree line for pinon and juniper trees on the same face of the same mountain. Add in the effects of latitude and you see that a tree line ranges from 0 ft. elevation in areas of Northern Quebec to 17,000 ft in the Andes of Bolivia.

Tree lines are much more dynamic and wavy and unpredictable than we thought, huh?

I am thankful for this first glimpse of a tree line, thankful Christian brought me to such heights. In seeing it with my own eyes, I find a place for tolerance to replace a rigid notion of what is that I had carried into that run. Maybe we just came up with a corollary (remember those from geometry?) about seeing the forest for the trees.

It is seeing the tree line for what it is – not a line at all.

It is seeing each other as clumps and groves with our unique way of being, beautiful growths within a 4-year old's painting, more human and more unified than our politics or media leads us to think.

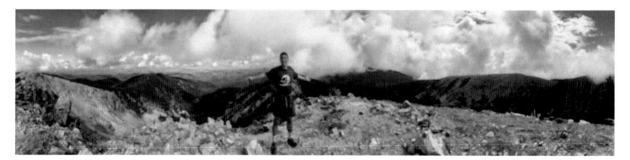

Action/Reflection:
Practice tolerance toward a group that you find hard to practice tolerance with/on. Reflect on how and why you find it hard to show tolerance for this group.

In the Dark No More

As a healer who has been doing my work in the dark, blind in a sense, today was a big day.

The visit was scheduled, not as a phone visit, but as my first Zoom visit since the pandemic began months ago. Usually, I see 50 patients in-person each week. During the last months, I have seen about this many - 50 patients total - in-person, with the vast majority of visits conducted as phone visits since the pandemic began.

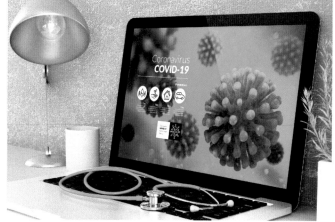

For someone who values that sacred space where the exam room creates a space where all other worries and commitments cease to matter for those 20 minutes, the only commitment being presence, this has been a big change. Put more bluntly it has been really hard for me. I am sure most of the patients and providers of the world feel similarly.

That sacred space is now replaced by a phone call with interruptions and multi-tasking, my kids often seeking daddy's attention as I sit in my home office (e.g. living room couch). Not being able to see people in these visits during COVID further dehumanizes the time together.

I signed on, not believing this was happening, but hoping I wasn't about to hear an alarm clock that would wake me from a pleasant dream.

In a touch-less, feet apart, face-covered-with-masks reality, I was about to get closer to the people I work with as a physician, the people who teach me about healing. I hoped this would re-create the sacred space I have been so missing.

When the visit started, Ms. Armijo *(name changed to protect patient confidentiality)* couldn't get the visual aspect on her tablet to work.

"Geez. I knew this was too good to be true," I mumbled to myself. I think it was just life's way of building the suspense, doing what all movie directors and novelists do so well. Make 'em wait for the good stuff. Then suddenly she was there, smiling at me. And I was able to smile back. No face masks to spoil the moment!

I really did not expect the rush of emotions that rushed and gushed in those next moments.

Here's a decent recap of them put into words:

Wow!

I can't believe this! I can see her and she can see me.

When I say, "I am really glad to have the chance to see you for this visit," I won't have to make a silly joke about what "see" means anymore.

I knew I was missing something big these last months, but wow, I didn't realize how much the human connection was lost in these phone call visits.

Warmth. Connection. Healing.

Healing of a great chasm created by 5 months of practicing medicine blindfolded.

Sacred space

Wow!

In that visit, and in the few I have done since then, I take time to ask the person to show me something about their life that I would never get to see, never be able to fully appreciate if the visit was done in a clinic.

Ms. Armijo chose to show me her service dog that has been such a big part of her healing journey. I licked the screen, an appropriate dog greeting. In exchange, I share something on my end – the garden, a picture, etc. Two humans just trying to find real connection in a virtual world.

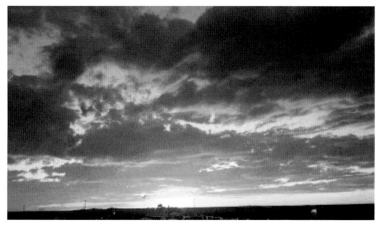

Appreciate these small moments today, tomorrow and next week. Those moments where the sacred spaces in your life suddenly return. Maybe not in quite the same form as they would have pre-pandemic, but good enough to make your heart skip a beat, for gratitude to grow. Reminding us all that the sacred spaces are still much closer to us than we think or see when in the dark. May light similarly shine your way today! May your own light be the illumination.

Action/Reflection:
Write about a moment you have had recently that was a "in the dark no more" experience.

Going to a Special Place

This week's piece is a chance for you to create space for yourself, maybe here at the end of a long week and maybe on a Monday morning when you see this.

You will need a few items for this exercise - do not pass
GO if you have not collected the following:

Ten minutes for yourself
A piece of paper
One of your favorite writing utensils

We are going to start with a meditation, and you can choose to do this either by reading the script below or by listening to the meditation below. Big choice. Go with your gut on this one:

Meditation - *audio version* - https.youtu.be/wdrytOwQ
Meditation - *written version*

Find a nice space, indoor or outdoor and get into a comfortable position, one free of pain. If possible, find a position where your feet are on the floor, where you are sitting tall, extending each of those vertebrae to their greatest height. Let those vertebrae breathe life into your body!

Once you have the position that feels good, just sit with that for a minute. Start to slow down the mind as the heart and your emotional/spiritual self takes over command of the ship.

Now, in a completely different place than you were a few minutes ago, you are ready for a journey.

Take some nice, slow, deep, rejuvenating breaths.
- Air in, deep into the recesses of those lungs, into the abdomen.
- Air out, expelling all that does not serve.

Take as much time as you need here, enjoying the state of being, the state of breathing.. This isyour time, and no one is rushing you through it.

Smile, and relax those face muscles. Smile at life, smile at the moment, smile at something thathas made you smile earlier today. Smile at all of your loved ones.

Now, with eyes gently closing, take yourself to a special place, a place that you have not been able to visit because of the pandemic. Take yourself to that place right now. Smell the fragrances this place brings to mind. Touch the things around you. Listen to the noises of this special place. Feel the energy around you. Sit with this and enjoy being and breathing in this special place for a minute or two.

Let's invite one person to enjoy this space with you. Maybe a person who, like this special place, you have not been able to see due to the pandemic. Or maybe someone that comes to mind when you think of this special place.

Invite them to join you. If you are at a beach, they are not sitting beside you in the soft sand. If you are hiking a forest or a favorite trail, they walk in stride with you. If you are in a place of prayer or meditation, they are praying/meditating next to you.

Enjoy this person's warmth and presence, as you both soak in this special moment together.

Take your time here. This is your time and the clock has stopped ticking. Your heart is now the only beat of time present, and it is set to "timeless" mode.

When you are ready, a few more deep, rejuvenating breaths and then open those 2 eyes to join the 3rd eye that is wide open at this point.

Paper and favorite writing utensil in hand, you are now going to write a hand-written letter to that person who joined you in the meditation. You are filled with healing energy and the writing itself is furthering your healing. There is something about writing on paper that reveals ourselves in a way that typing onto a phone or computer simply cannot. As you write, think of how this letter is going to brighten the person's day. Think of how you are going to deliver it. Write in joy! Deliver the letter within the next week.

Repeat as needed.

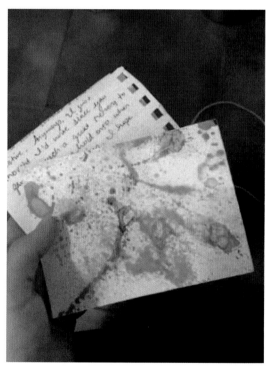

Action/Reflection:
Write the letter described above and deliver it within the next week.

After posting this piece, Veronica Hutchison, an amazing mentee of mine, writes the following along with the picture above.: "Just listened to your newest Writing to Heal meditation. I found this funky envelope that I made at a "self care" Native Health Initiative event. Perfect for this letter!"

Sacred Play and Imaginary Escapes

Hope things go back to normal soon."

That was the text I received from a friend yesterday. It struck me in reading those words that I have stopped thinking or worrying about the end of the pandemic. In those first months, absolutely. Daily thoughts of getting back to normal life. Now, out of self-preservation and a renewed sense of life's sacredness, I have turned to making the most of each day, not wasting a moment of living spending time trying to beg normal to reappear.

My response was simply, Yep!!But let's make the most of each day until then." And in that spirit, I want to share two stories that remind us to find joy, creativity, sacred play, even imaginary escape as tools for thriving in our new normal. Enjoy.

The Teacher Has Arrived

Our house is a weird place these days. We don't own a TV, our children don't have phones, and we are as close to screen-free as a modern day family could be. But now? Now, we are people zoomed in to our classes and work, zoned out from each other and the world beyond our square inches of screen space. We have a 7th, 4th and 1st grader and all of them have adapted well to this online life.

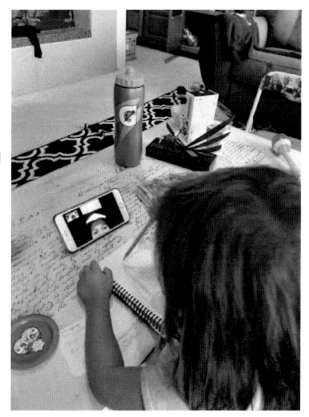

Our 2 year-old Sihasin has taken in this sudden change, and it is interesting to see her interpretation of this virtual world. Dad, do you have another meeting?she will ask the second I open my computer. Dad, are you going to your office anytime she senses that I am about to start a work session. Office, as she has figured out, is a very loose term and could apply to garage, porch, kitchen, living room, etc. Office dress, as she and her siblings have observed,ranges from tank

Action shot of little one at "school" with Ms. B

tops to running shirts to sleepwear to an occasional collared shirt.

Well, Sihasin voiced that she wanted to go to school just like everyone else. She was feeling left out, not having a screen of her own to stare into. So Nizhoni, our oldest devised a plan. On times when she was not in school, she would sneak upstairs, put on a disguise, and become the teacher for Sihasin. Let me explain that "disguise" in this context means simply changing 1-2 things about appearance. I asked Nizhoni if she uses a different voice as teacher, and she gave me a look. Dad, that really isn't necessary. I use my normal voice and I still don't think she knows it is me."

So, Teacher Nizhoni broadcasts from upstairs to Student Sihasin who we get onto a tablet downstairs. Teacher Nizhoni goes by Miss B"and gives her choices. Do you want to do music or dance today. Usually, the class is quite short as Student Sihasin loses interest and simply walks away from the screen. No good bye"or I have to go now" but just a departure to signal that this class session has ended. Teacher Nizhoni is quite understanding.

Pics of, in order of appearance, Teacher Nizhoni and (Regular) Nizhoni

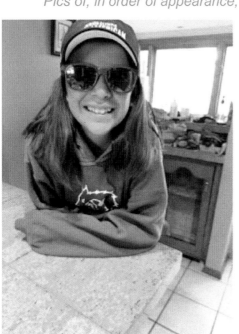
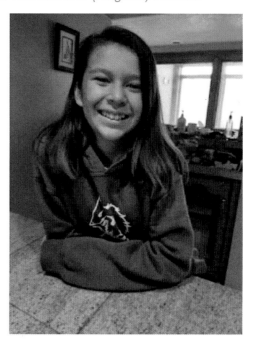

A Breathe of Fresh Air is All We Need

We were a tired group of physicians, immersed in sickness, loneliness, COVIDness as we cared for patients at UNM Hospital. The week had worn us down, taking out our zip and pep and replaced it with argghhh. I think someone mentioned something about fresh air in a figurative sense, but I suddenly realized that real fresh air was exactly the antidote. With inertia of hospital work and an indoor existence the entire week working against us, I was able to coax everyone to come outside with me. I had tried multiple times previously in the week to get us outside, failing each time. Inertia and a huge work load will do that. This time, I think the combination of me using my best attempt at an authoritative voice plus the presence of argghhh" made the group start to warm up to the idea of a few minutes outside.

We found a nice place of shade on a beautiful late May afternoon and suddenly we were transformed. The grass felt so good, so real. The hospital walls now dissolved, we were free in mind and spirit. Free from work. Free from the burden of so much hardship that was our patients' reality. Free from ourselves. Spontaneously, the crew starting talking about how incredible it felt to be outside. How it surprised them how quickly they felt rejuvenated by shade, breeze, birds, grass and all that now embraced our senses.

The power of fresh air and simple escapes. From argghhh"to this pic below in a matter of minutes.

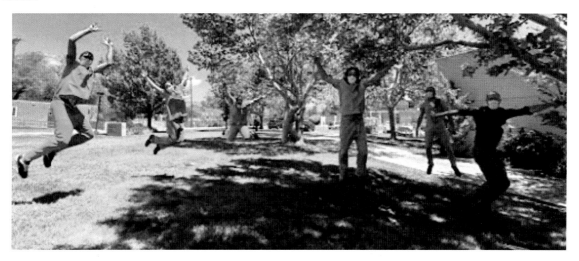

May you find joy,creativity, sacred play, even imaginary escape as tools for thriving in our new normal. Practice daily. Titrate dose upward if needed. Enjoy the silly moments along the way.

Action/Reflection:
Try out sacred play and/or an imaginary escape this week. This is best done from your desk at work, when driving a car, and in other mundane parts of the week.

Connection

We had turned to leave, the ICU machines and monitors beeping their goodbyes.

Working at the University of New Mexico's Hospital as a family physician, I had come to visit this patient with a colleague who is a physician assistant upon the request of the ICU team.

Our patient, Ms. Armijo, an elderly woman who'd been hospitalized in critical condition after emergency abdominal surgery for abdominal pain called out after us. "You know, the thing I am really worried about is being all alone."

As we turned around, and I saw Ms. Armijo's fright amidst her frail, failing body.

I had thought that our lengthy, pathology-driven questioning had covered all of the bases pretty thoroughly. Where do you hurt.?How do you hurt. Are the pain meds working for you?

Now, frozen in mid-stride by her question, I realized that we had neglected the most important thing: Connectedness.

COVID had forced our hospital to adopt a no-visitors policy. On every floor, the hand-holding and bedside banter that partners, siblings, neighbors and coworkers normally lavish on hospital patients was replaced by a sickening silence. Even I, a family physician, couldn't visit my own patients who'd been hospitalized or sent to skilled nursing facilities due to COVID.

Imagine yourself in that ICU bed. Scared for your life, feeling so weak that you cannot even lift a spoon to your mouth--and suffering all of this alone, without the comfort of your loved ones at your side.

This was the situation Ms. Armijo was facing. Not only that, she didn't even have her connection to her family and the outside world with her cell phone missing. No wonder she was distraught!

Our team went back to her bedside. This time we did the listening, not the talking.

"I have no idea what happened to my cell phone in all of this," she started. "Have you been able to talk with your sister and family?" I asked. "No, and that's what I am really worried about. My sister who takes care of me and she must be going crazy not knowing how I am doing. Sitting here, I don't think they even know if I made it out of surgery alive. If it weren't for the pandemic, they would be sitting right here by my side.'"

I was being taught, the physician as the student, my patient Ms. Armijo as my teacher.

"Thank you for sharing," was all I could muster.

"This is not a 'no news is good news' scenario for them," she added.

Listening to her speak, both what was spoken and lay in the pauses and expressions, I was not ashamed but more eager to be her student. To me, it felt like a direct, visceral reminder [or some such] that asking Ms. Armijo about her sense of connectedness, or otherwise, was as important as probing into her abdominal pain and lab results. We were being taught that you cannot have full health or healing if you're disconnected from those you love.

I've started to realize that connectedness can actually be considered as yet another vital sign--as important, in its way, as any heart rhythm or puff of breath.

And in these extraordinarily difficult times, loneliness can almost be considered a new medical condition, one affecting close to 100% of our hospitalized patients, one requiring its own treatment plan. This was true, I realized, not only for Ms. Armijo but for all of our hospitalized and nursing facility patients.

The phone was found by her family, discarded in the chaos that led to her ambulance ride to the hospital. Over the next few hours, with painstaking effort, it was delivered to the hospital - passed like a hot potato to the security guard at curbside, then to a nurse courier, past the badge-access checkpoints and, finally, safely into the hands of Ms. Armijo.

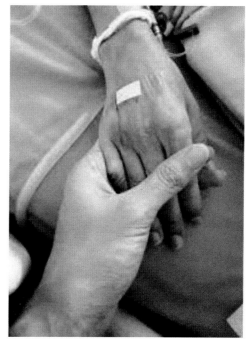

Her body still had a long way to go in terms of healing. But she was now connected back into her world, her support system.

Heading to the next patient on our list, we all knew which question we would ask first. It would not be about pain level, appetite, or bowel movements. Those would wait for later. First question would be simply, How can we help connect you to those you love?"

Action/Reflection:
Write about how challenges you have had in connecting with others and how connection has changed for you during the pandemic.

Signs of Change

Can things really change??

Can our country find a way to admit systemic racism and then do the hard work to undue it??

Can we begin to live with our Earth, ending our suicidal quest to dominate it??

Will we begin to honor the Indigenous Peoples of this land, reversing their second-class status in a land that is their own.

Well, I can't honestly answer all of these questions with a positive answer. At least not with confidence. But I can see some signs that make me hopeful. I want to share two of those with you. Example 1:: U.S. Forest Service

My family thought about places to get away and enjoy a hike. The outdoors seem to be one place where the pandemic loses its grasp over us. Aside from a piece of fabric covering the face's mid-section, you almost can forget about words like "feet apart""and "Zoom".

With fatherly skill, I quickly steered the conversation toward Wheeler Peak, my selfish choice for our hike. Our tallest mountain in NM at 13,147 feet, I had wanted to climb this for many years. We looked up the hike and found that, at that moment, the trails in that area were closed. Reading further, they were closed due to traditional ceremonies of the Taos Pueblo.

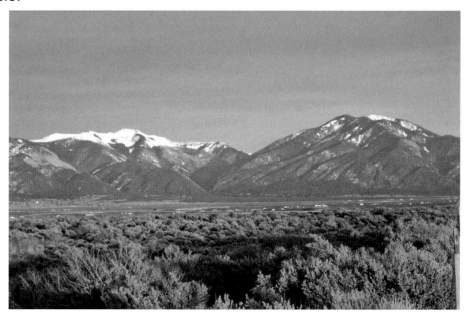

Carson Forest Supervisor, James Duran stated,

"It's important that the Carson National Forest works to support local traditional communities to continue a traditional way of life that makes the culture of Northern New Mexico so rich and truly unique. We appreciate the public's patience and willingness to support our local tribal communities in maintaining long standing connections to these mountains during this unique period."

YESSSSS!!!!!!!!!!!!!!

Many of us, myself included, may never have associated public lands and the National Park System as anything beyond an attempt to conserve and preserve the natural beauty of our country. But Indigenous communities have a very different history with the creation of such lands.

Just as land was stolen from these people since the arrival of Europeans, conservation efforts simply provided another avenue to trample over these same communities. As Marcus Colchester writes, "National parks, pioneered in the United States, denied indigenous peoples rights, evicted them from their homelands, and provoked long-term social conflict. This model of conservation became central to conservation policy worldwide.""

Making the position of the Carson Forest even more important is the context of Taos Pueblo and the U.S. Forest Service. Just a few miles away from Wheeler Peak is Blue Lake, known to the Taos Pueblo as Ba Whyea, a sacred site to that Tribe used for many traditional ceremonies.

In the name of conservation, the U.S. government appropriated Blue Lake and the surrounding area and placed it under the control of the Forest Service. The Equivalent of The Vatican being taken away from Catholics, Mecca confiscated from Muslims. These thefts usually came without consultation with Indigenous communities. The struggle by Taos Pueblo to regain control of Blue Lake similar to Standing Rock in 2016, represented Indigenous struggles for religious freedom and the protection of sacred sites.

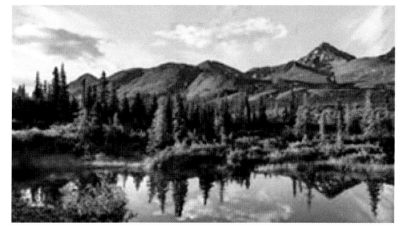

(After 64 years of protest, appeal, and lobbying by Taos leaders and their supporters, Blue Lake was restored to the Pueblo in 1970).

So, to see the Forest Service now working as a protector, not a threat to Taos Pueblo is a victory for all of us. To see words acknowledging that traditional ways are what make our land unique is incredible in a land that has largely ignored and""othered""Indigenous ways at best, often working explicitly to eradicate them completely. (Kill the Indian, Save the Man" policy of the U.S. Boarding Schools, for example).

Example 2: Princeton University

No, I was not about to take my family on a trip to New Jersey. "Kids, jump in the car. We are heading to audit a weekend course at an Ivy League institution."" Not quite.

But September 2nd letter by Princeton's president Christopher Eisgruber to acknowledge systemic racism caught my eye.

"Racism and the damage it does to people of color nevertheless persist at Princeton as in our society, sometimes by conscious intention but more often through unexamined assumptions and stereotypes, ignorance or insensitivity, and the systemic legacy of past decisions and policies. Race-based inequities in America's health care, policing, education, and employment systems affect profoundly the lives of our staff, students, and faculty of color.

Racist assumptions from the past also remain embedded in structures of the University itself. For example, Princeton inherits from earlier generations at least nine departments and programs organized around European languages and culture, but only a single, relatively small program in African studies."

YESSSSS!!!!!!!!

Coming from an institution that represents power and privilege, this divergence from the default - finding ways to justify unjust systems that serve to benefit that person/group speaking - is refreshing. It is healing. It is needed.

So, back to those initial questions, I can say that I have some hope that I can be a part of making real change happen. That is the only place any of us can start – acknowledging our own responsibility to pave a different road for our own lives, our own words, our own actions. We can be transformed just like the Forest Service and Princeton University to stand for undoing racism and a new way of treating each of Creator's beautiful creations, land/air/animals included.

Healing awaits us, my brothers and sisters.

Action/Reflection:

Land acknowledgments are an example of signs of change, and have become more present since the murder of George Floyd. Write your own personal Land Acknowledgment this week, reflecting on the original inhabitants of the land on which you reside.

The Ever-Present Presence of the Present

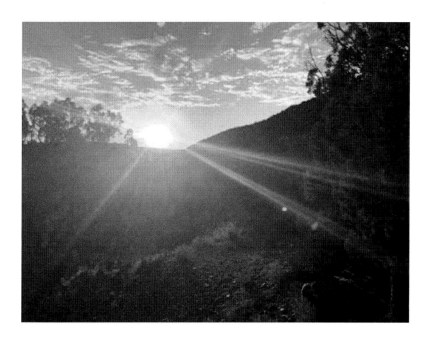

The ever-present

Presence

> *of the*

Present

> *a*

Present

> *Gifted to those seeking its warm*
>
> *embrace*
>
> *Remedy for dis-ease*
>
> *Cure for living in worlds*
>
> *"Has been"*
>
> *"What was"*
>
> *"Yet-to-come"*

The ever-present

Presence

   of the

Present

   Is our natural state

   Known well to little ones and wise elders

   Sought by those in between (if they even care to seek)

   Like all things valuable, it can't be captured by smartphone, thumb drive, DVR

The ever-present

Presence

   of the

Present

   a

Present

   That offers itself to us at this precious moment

   And next hour

   And all of tomorrow

   Fear not as you reach to greet its embrace

Note: This piece brought me back to the second piece in this *Writing to Heal blog, a prose piece about the Superpower of Being Present. Feel free to revisit that piece!

*https://writingtoheal1.blogspot.com/2020/04/the-superpower-of-being-pesent.html/

Gháájí': New Year, New You

Renewal

As full moon lights the sky,

Gháájí', the Navajo New Year is celebrated.

A chance for all of us five-fingered people to breathe deep

give thanks renew

vows to self

life

each other

Leaves brighten to hues not seen since 2019019 Melons, squash, apples reaching maturity after months of growing pains.

Mornings crisp with scents of Green Chile wafting olfactory goodness your way. Cinnamon, pumpkin and other flavors soon to come.

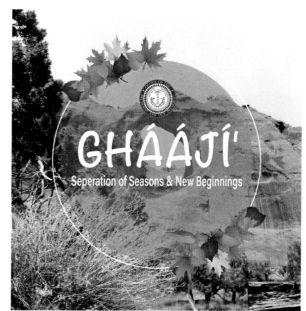

What do you want the new year to look like?
What do you want the new you to look like?
What do you need to leave behind in the year that was?
What must be cultivated in the year to come?
Beyond the seeds themselves,
How will you water and fertilize and nurture those seeds you plant?
Where do you want to start?

Action/Reflection:

Take some time this week to breathe deep,
get out the Crayolas, canvas, journal, etc. and begin to dream/sketch/write of an area in your life where you want to create a "new you".

October 7, 2020

Bass and Treble

Way back when, humans listened to music without Spotify, Air Pods, smart phones, and blue teeth/tooths.

In those B.S.P. (Before Smart Phones) days, people would actually get off their *tooshies* (medical term for gluteal area) and walk over to a thing called a stereo to adjust the sound using something called an equalizer. Crazy huh??Millennials reading this are already distractedly Googling all of this to verify I am not spinning tall tales.

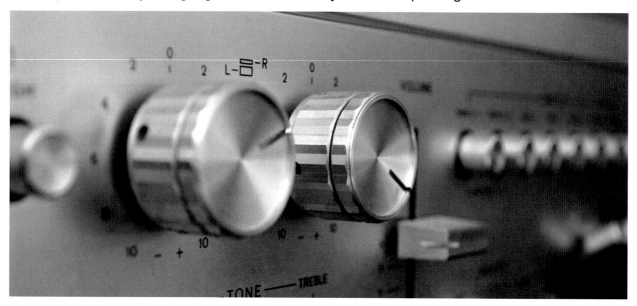

Let's use the equalizer analogy as we consider what music we play for ourselves today. Treble represents the positive in life – the beautiful moments of each day, the practice of gratitude and the people and experiences that make us grateful. All that sustains us will be treble.

Bass, meanwhile, represents the negative – things that stress us, things that cause us to worry, fear, and which bring on anxiety.

Yes, life does give us a starting material for the music we hear, but it is our decision of how we adjust the equalizer that makes the difference between symphony and cacophony. "Woe is me"is not a reflection of the orchestra, but is a reflection of that person's inability to lower the bass so that treble can ring.

And if treble weren't easy to tune up, the majority of media even exist. Regurgitating the same bad news, knowing humans will consume it over and over and over. In those rare cases of treble amongst so much bass, you would never hear a feel good"story repeated one day to the next on the 10 pm news.

"Now to follow up on that incredible tale of the boy who raised $10,000 for his classmate with cancer from yesterday. We thought we would take another look at this tale since we felt it was so important for our city."

Nope. But crime, natural disasters, political squabbling attract attention day after day. I think our own internal news feed"plays out similarly. Much easier to regurgitate and perseverate on the bass in our lives.

My friends, play with the equalizer today. Play with that innate ability to attune to treble and let the positive dictate your thoughts and actions. Bass will still be there, but it will exist in balance with, and in the context of the treble sound. You might even appreciate new and more constructive angles on the bass sounds by not focusing on them.

Today, life will not give us treble or bass. No, today we get to choose how to manipulate the equalizer and make music out of the sounds that life presents.

A simple exercise for those interested in tuning their equalizer:
Write down 3 things that have most bothered/worried you in the last week. These are your bass.

Now, take those 3 things and come up with the opposite statement. Ex., "I am worried about my grandmother's health becomes. I am grateful to have my grandmother in my life.""

Today, as you go about the day, when you find yourself beginning to think in "bass", simply adjust the equalizer and turn that worry into its "treble" opposite.

Repeat as needed.

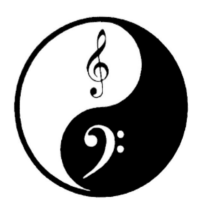

Action/Reflection:
Do the exercise above.

Write your own piece on "bass and treble" and feel free to include your insights from the exercise above.

Mask Up!

I wear a mask

Some might label me a sheep

Yes, proudly I am

In fact, it is something called herd immunity*

Proudly part of the herd

Baah' baah'

I wear a mask.

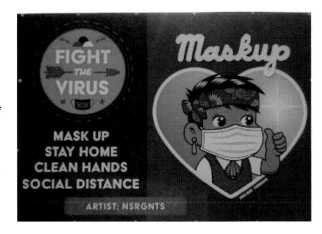

Even as a doc, I can't cite you the risk level as another person passes

But I wear the mask to show respect for their life, their health, and their family at home

And yes, for myself and my family at home as well

I wear a mask

Not any more as a political statement than

getting a flu shot

flushing the toilet

or picking up my dog's poop

I wear it because it is the right thing to do as a member of a larger community that relies on me to make the right decision

I wear it because I don't want to see communities of color suffer any further in this pandemic

I don't want anyone to suffer

I wear a mask

Believing in science

I wear a mask and ask that you do the same Why?

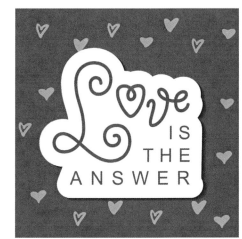

Because you are too important not to be here because of COVID

I wear a mask and ask that you do the same

Why?

Because you are too important not to be here because of COVID

Ditto for those in your family

Ditto for those you might infect

I wear a mask and ask that you do the same

Because it is a statement of love for your community

Because together we can bring reason, humanity, and caring for each other back into this polarized, angry shouting match we find ourselves in

Because we are together in this herd called humanity

Baah' baah'

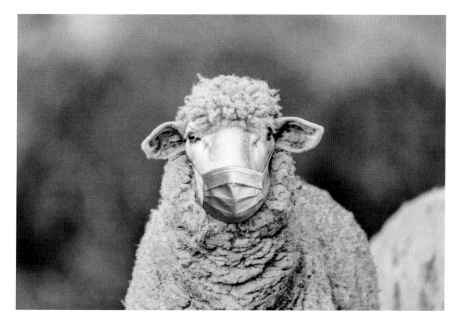

**As a professor in population health, I need to clarify that herd immunity is not quite the same as wearing a mask. Herd immunity is the idea that if enough people are immunized, the herd as a whole is protected. But in this case, I couldn't resist the poetic connection between sheep...herd...herd immunity.
This blog is an escape from my academic life, after all :)*

Action/Reflection:
What does the facemask represent for you in the pandemic? Write about it.

Explosion

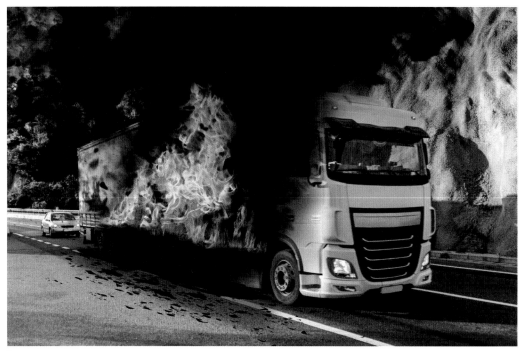

Explosion

Flames tenaciously, menacingly bursting upward

The truck sat in the middle of the road, consumed by the fiery uproar

Its driver remained in the vehicle

Smoke signaled impending doom

Explosion

Of humanity rushing from their vehicles

Thirty or more sprinted in superhero form toward the vehicle

Using their strength, wits, and first responder skills to

> *pry open passenger door*
>
> *pry hope from despair*
>
> *pry life from death's grasp*

We worked in harmony like ants bringing an injured comrade back to the colony,

Successfully bringing the driver out safely,

Stopping traffic and all that we might have been rushing to do.

No one cared about political affiliation, where you worshipped, views on abortion, immigration status, bank account balance, color of skin, educational status, sexual orientation.

All unimportant.

We were unified in saving a life.

We were connected in a struggle to

> *pry open passenger door*
>
> *pry hope from despair*
>
> *pry life from death's grasp*

We needed each other.

Why can't we similarly unify, dropping everything that divides to find our mutuality, our common bonds on the other fiery emergencies of this moment?

Systemic Racism that threatens to burn us to a crisp.

A virus that laughs through its flames as politics infect public health to the detriment of us all.

Let us need each other more

Let us connect with each other's humanity

Ignore the bumper stickers on the car

See the beautiful being who sits amidst flames within

Fire that threatens both of you

> *all of us*
>
> *Act accordingly*
>
> *Explosion of love*
>
> *Explosion of love*
>
> *Explosion of love*

Action/Reflection:
Write about a moment where your witnessed an "explosion of love" in the past week.

Jump!

Like a good dad, when my kids talk I listen.

"Dad, we want a trampoline."

My mind went where most parents' minds go when expensive, potentially dangerous requests are made from our well-intentioned little ones.

Which neighbor has a trampoline so that I can fulfill this request, I pondered.

Luckily, I could answer the question. A lovely neighbor does indeed have one of these jumping, bouncing polypropylene sandboxes with springs. And in good condition. And with netting to make me feel safer as a parent.

So, after gaining permission to jump, we headed over to try it out.

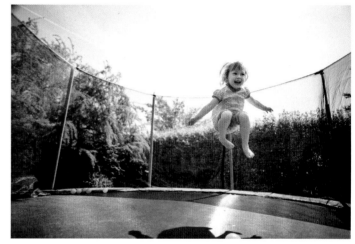

Our three oldest got right to jumping. No hesitation. Barely a "Thank you for letting us invade your yard and use your trampoline for our dad who is too cheap to buy us one."

Our smallest watched for a few moments, trying to figure this out. Clearly, she had second thoughts. Has she read the Pediatrics guidelines around injury risks from such devices?

I picked her up and placed her on the springy surface.

Her look back to me communicated a strong skepticism.

Dear, you jump up and then have fun falling down."

In her mind: "Fall. Falling down. That means getting hurt, boo-boos, ouchies, band-aids."

Despite my pleading, I couldn't convince her that this was a safe place to jump and fall. I carried her off the trampoline.

We don't jump because we are afraid to fall.

We don't take that leap because of the security of feeling our feet on the ground.

We miss the exhilaration of being airborne because we are so focused on what happens when we come down.

Fear of failure holds us back from envisioning the heights we can reach.

Focusing on past "ouchies" and falls keeps us from jumping ahead.

Trauma and scars from hitting the ground in the past trip us up in the present, both keeping us from jumping and putting us into a "fall mindset"

So much so that when a trampoline moment presents itself, with possibilities of reaching superhero heights, we turn around and ask to get off without having taken a jump.

Even when trampoline moments ask us to suspend our beliefs around falling, ask us to re-consider the equation falling = failing, it is still tempting to back away without ever going airborne.

Excited to where you all take this analogy, how you choose to finish the piece…

Excited to hear whether this piece helps you jump!

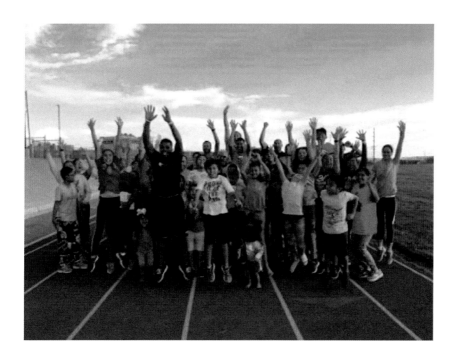

Action/Reflection:
Try "jumping" this week, going for something that you might otherwise talk yourself out of out of fear of falling.

A Vision for Undoing Racism + Achieving Equity in Health

Thirty-three times I have written.

In gratitude.

In confidence that we can turn our world toward hope and healing.

Of our planet. Of ourselves. Of our communities.

This week, I want to focus on someone else's writing.

A long time ago, back in October when COVID numbers were low, we were asked to give a keynote address at the New Mexico Public Health Association (NMPHA) conference on racism and health equity. Adults speaking to adults.

It seemed like a perfect moment to get creative and bring youth voices into the conversation.

So, we asked young leaders from our Native Health Initiative partnership to meet at Robinson Park on a pandemic Sunday. Bring an open heart and dress in a way that reflects your cultures. No other instructions.

We sat beneath a tree. Air was calm, birds chirped their hellos.

The youth began to write, speaking to their experiences of what they had to tell the world on undoing racism, to working toward equity in health. They spoke about not being listened to enough by the adult world.

Their voices were captured on film, with my brother leading the way on the videography side of things. I had contributed the concept for the film, but the youth wrote all of their own lines.

Hip hop culture, both in the art and the music would provide the backdrop for the film.

The conversations were interesting as we moved from one location to another.

"Does mentioning this take away from our work, implying that despite the handicap of being young, that we still made big things happen?" they discussed.

Does focusing on healthcare miss the larger picture of what allows people to have health?

What does a healthy education system look like?

What does a healthy food system mean??

What does a healthy neighborhood feel like??

Without further ado, I would like to present their vision, their answers. This film was premiered at that NMPHA conference, saved as the last part of the address.

Youth speaking. Adults listening.

Watch the 2 minute film by visiting - https://vimeo.com/46407525353

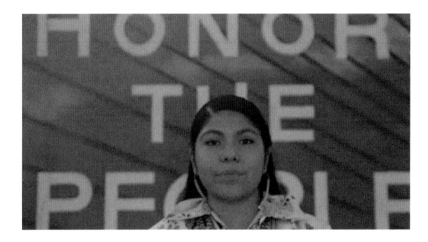

After the film showed, Emelia spoke and we put up the last slide, to make sure everyone had heard their call to action:

Call to action to NMPHA from our youth

1) Start with yourselves and your friends – keep each other accountable
2) Decolonize and localize our food systems
3) Don't minimize racism – accept it and do your part to reverse it
4) Support us and trust youth to lead the way

Action/Reflection:
How can you create more space for youth to lead? Answer through action!!

Writing to Heal: The 45-Word Edition

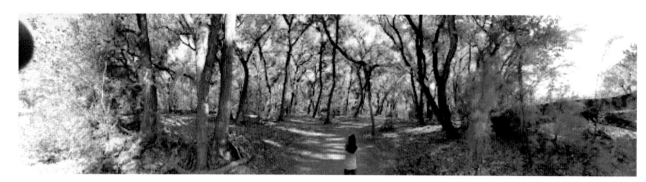

Calm

Peace

Tranquility

Breathe them in, slow and deep

Calm

Peace

Tranquility

Embrace your antidote

44

COVID Craze

Virtual Daze

Dizzying Maze

Calm fears with gratitude

Peace

Tranquility your new attitude

Breathe them in, slow and deep

Grow your own healing

If necessary, use words.

Action/Reflection:

This week, I wanted to play with a self-imposed challenge: what can I say in 50 words or less that is meaningful around the climate where election and COVID spike has everything stirred up. Take the challenge yourself - 50 words or less 😊

Bowls Into Cabinets

How does a clean bowl get put back into the cabinets?

Not a trick question, but a real dilemma if you are a little one.

Dwarfed by the imposing height of the cabinets, my kiddos huddled to discuss. Eavesdropping, here is what I heard,

Small legs.

Big cabinets.

Clean bowls.

Should we just go play?

I need to go potty.

Like any respectable adult, I tried to re-focus my mind on real things. Quickly move on from this frivolity to things adults should be thinking about.

What shirt to re-wear for work from the couch today? Pajama pants again?

How to balance personal wellness and being up-to-date in my pandemic news consumption today?

Why aren't there any clean bowls in the cabinet?

Should we just go play?

I need to go potty.

About a week later, not intending to get to the bottom of the mystery, I did just that. Catching a glimpse of the children shuttling clean bowls to empty cabinets, I snuck with fatherly deftness around the kitchen's perimeters.

Channeling my inner James Bond, looking over my shoulders for any sign of "bad guys", I crouched low.

Ouch. A bit too low.

Should have stretched out before trying that.

Here is what I saw.:

When life gives you imposing challenges today and in these next weeks, become the child you still are. Throw away ego and figure out who it is around you who can help you reach the cabinets.

As COVID roars, the cabinets seem higher than normal, the kitchen is lonely, and the bowls are staring at you. In those moments, become a little one again. Reach out, reach up for the support you need. Think about friends, family, neighbors who might be reaching for the cabinet, and offer a hand before they ask.

And finally, give in to those two nagging thoughts we adults so carefully suppress:

Should we just go play?

I need to go potty.

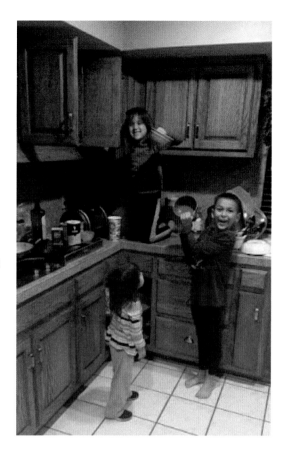

Gratitude

Gratitude

Grows with slowing down, stillness

Gratitude

Knows the nooks and crannies of our soul, landing gently like Sandhill Crane upon

Fertile

Feeding ground.

Flows

    Over

    Into

        the places trampled upon by 2020

        setting them

        anew

        alive

        awakened.

This week of thanks

    giving

    gave me a chance to hear beautiful answers to question

"What does gratitude sound, feel (heart and hands), smell, and look like for you??"

Enjoy the feast as you scribe your own answers and share them with loved ones!

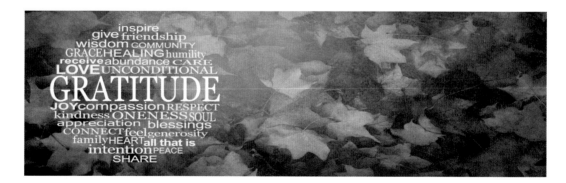

I am grateful for the eyes,

the eyes of the heart,

as they look at the beauty within

and the beauty not often seen in all of life.

I am grateful for the hands,

the hands that serve others,

as they reach out to lift others up and push them gently to positivity and inspiration.

I am grateful for the ears,

the ears that listen,

as they hear the laughter of the child, a parent's cry, a partner mourning,

and Creator's way to live in happiness.

Eyes of the heart,

Hands that serve others,

Ears that listen,

all working together to make one

feel loved

give love

and not lose their way with Living in Love, Loving in Life.

– Shannon

Effortless breath; birds singing as if it was spring; a smile for no apparent reason. Sun rise and set—one thing we can count on.

Still breathing.

-Amy

What does gratitude sound like?

 Thank you… You're welcome

What does gratitude feel like?

 In your heart: peace…safety…love

 In your hands: sharing…showing…building

What does gratitude smell like?

 Cut grass…fallen leaves…rain

What does gratitude look like?

 Birds flying in unison…dogs sleeping…warm fire pit

-Michael

Gratitude for me is ubiquitous.

It is in the rising of the sun

and the rising of the moon

and

it is observing the values you have

strived to live by reflected back by

your children and grandchildren.

-Allan

Delicately waking up to the aromas of love and lemon pepper

Stretching to the blessings

High flying the transitioned

Nature is shut down but there are genealogical trees swaying, growing and smiling green leaves of joy in the room we live

Standing on the mountains of our ancestors

Gazing at each gift amongst the abode

Beholden the Creator!

Fully seasoned with warmth, comfort, paprika, life and a dash of salt

Family recipes ready to consume

Imbibing the earth's hydrogen, hydrogen, and oxygen

Everyone safely encompassed in these four walls

Beholden the Creator!

Deeply,

Inhaling a soul full of gratitude

For there is nothing more to want

Thankful

-Danielle

Action/Reflection:

Create a quite space and place this week to immerse yourself in gratitude. Share what you experience in this exercise with someone close to you.

Drift

trail

turned

to

snowy

    drift I did

into a world not virtual

into a space immaculate

into myself

drift today into your own not-virtual

        immaculate space

      dare to unplug from all of the noise

    sounds that silence the lullaby that trail of life is wafting your way

drift far away, to dreams and ancestors and all that fills your cup

drift to yourself

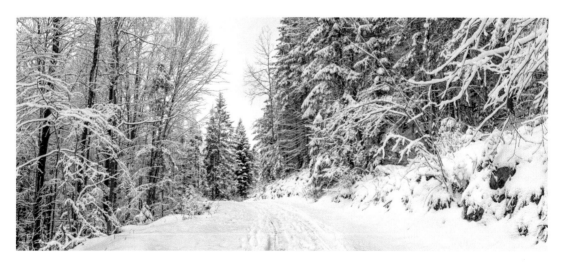

Special thanks to Mother Nature and the snow she provided somewhat unexpectedly last week for us in New Mexico.

Vaccinating Despair, Injecting Hope

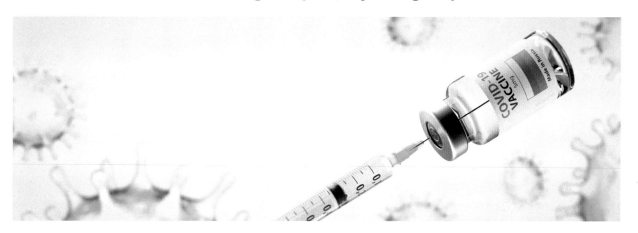

Vaccinating despair

Immunizing against virus

and

viral fear and isolation

Inoculating resilience

Injecting hope

Inspiring immune response

and

infectious optimism

I had some other thoughts for this week's piece, but the energy brought on by the arrival of a vaccine has truly been infectious. I couldn't ignore it. As a writer, I know that you speak to the moment. It might not be there next week. That has been my guide through this blog's existence.

I asked a group of first graders this morning about what they were going to do over winter break. Okay, okay - I actually asked them what healthy things they were going to do over break. A few students answered that question with "I think we need to get back to going to school. Some answered with a question of their own, "When is this going to be over?"

I agree with these 6 year- olds that it would be great for our health and wellness to get back to a normal existence. And while I don't have an answer for where/when the finish line is of this endurance challenge, it is a wonderful place that we find ourselves this week as the first COVID vaccines are given.

The vaccine is a holiday present delivered with dry ice and stored at negative 70 degree Celsius. Batteries sold separately. Restrictions apply. Not available in all 50 states...yeah, we know the verbiage of latest, greatest holiday gifts all too well.

PlayStation move over, Pfizer move in. Asking partner "Can we afford this?" replaced by questioning health insurance, "Will you cover it?"

The vaccine is a small bit of light cracking through the end of the tunnel. Do you see it? Look closer. Squint if you need to.

The vaccine is a reason to smile, sigh and maybe even cause for tear ducts to open.

The vaccine is an invitation for all of us to move past despair and 2020 and all that we need to leave behind.

Let us roll up our sleeve and accept the injection of hope.

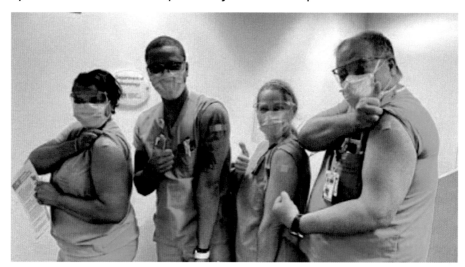

University of New Mexico's healthcare workers show off their "boo boos" on first day of vaccinations this week.

Action/Reflection:

When you think of moments of hope during the pandemic, what comes to mind? Write about this, and if you want to reflect on your thoughts when you first heard about the vaccine, go for it.

Shepherd's Journey

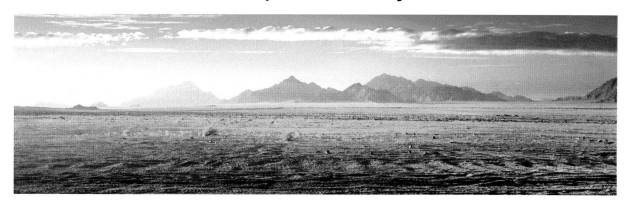

One day closer

One week closer

One month closer

The shepherd, tired and weak, shielded his eyes from the gusts of sand as he climbed yet another hill in the vast desert.

He did as he had done every day since setting out on this journey - peering as far he could into the distance ahead of him, he looked desperately for signs of the oasis that was his destination.

And like every day prior, his visioning led to disappointment, with nothing but endless sand in view. He walked on. Sheep bleating. Shepherd stick beating with a rhythmic thud on the desert sand.

Around mid-day, with sun scorching, a terrible gust of wind came blowing across the landscape. He could see it approaching from in front of him. Airborne tunnels of sand served as the trumpeters announcing the impending arrival of the king. In this case, the wind.

To this point, he had taken these moments head-on, not wanting to waste time in his quest for the oasis. But today, tired and weak, he made a different decision.
"I will not give the wind the satisfaction of slapping my face today."

With that, he stopped and turned away from the wind, so that he was facing toward where he had been on this journey.

To the sheep's and his surprise, he sat down.

Thud. Not a gentle landing.

He assumed a fetal position. And began to weep.

No one knows how much time passed, but a good while later, he awoke. The winds had battered his back and he noticed a stinging sensation over his spine. Still sitting, the shepherd uncurled from the fetal position, stretching his legs out in front of him. The wind has passed.

"I have beaten the wind today," he sighed.

He gazed upon the rolling desert over which he had traveled over the last days. And his mind began to wander.

Looking a good distance toward the horizon, he saw where he had been a day earlier. He smiled.

Squinting still further, he could see where he had been this same time last week. He smiled bigger.

And with his mind's eye, he looked further still, to where he had been exactly one month ago. You could now see his teeth with the smile.

"I am here. I can go on. My victory today is simply moving forward, one step at a time." These words appeared to him.

He rose, shook off sand, and awakened the sheep. "Such lazy animals," he thought with a chuckle, turning back to face his unknown destination.

His journey continued, but it was different now. There was hope, even joy as he took each step forward toward the oasis. Yes, tiredness as well.

And each day, around mid-day when the sun was scorching and even if there was no headwind, he would turn 180 degrees to whence he had come and say softly to himself and the sheep:

One day closer

One week closer

One month closer

Thank you for taking this healing journey with me.
May your path forward be one of joy and gratitude.
Make it so!

~~~~~~~~~~~~~~~

Gratitude and Acknowledgments

Writing to Heal, beginning in the first weeks of the project where it was word documents being sent by email to folks, has been about a community healing together.

Thank you to everyone that has supported me in your email responses, your reflections, your posts on the blog, and for your ways of supporting me to keep writing. A few people deserve special recognition in this realm. Thank you Shannon for sharing life with me and supporting this endeavor. Thank you kids! You gave daddy so much wisdom and humor to inspire me to write.

Then there are the folks who have supported me and this Writing to Heal project from day 1. Without you all, I might have stopped writing a long time ago. Thank you Amy, Valerie, Ted, Allan, Tonya, Michael, Ali, Solomon, Christine, Michael, Debie, and Tionna.

This book gave me the chance to share space with many creative people and for them I give thanks. Mallery Quetawki, one of my favorite artists who did the front cover. Hakim Bellamy, my brother whose poetry has a permanent place in my heart. David Rakel who has always supported me. One of my life mentors Freeman Hrabowski – you are a guide for my life.

Then there are beautiful people who contributed material for the book. Christian Gering, Joe Romero, Shannon Fleg, Tonya Covington, Randy Sabaque, Nehemiah Cionelo, Emelia Pino, Leah Lewis, Danielle Hopkins, Michael Nuttall, Amy Robinson, Veronica Hutchison and the Paint for Peace artists – thank you!

To Alex Paramo and Community Publishing, thank you for believing in me and supporting the book wholeheartedly. Buy local, including your publisher!

I give thanks to Creator for each moment on this earth.

About the Author

Anthony Fleg is a family medicine physician, a healer whose work is grounded in love, culture and community. He is from Baltimore, MD and has three younger brothers with familial roots in Germany, Poland and Russia.

Anthony lives in Albuquerque, NM with his wife Shannon, a Dine' (Navajo) woman who guides him in life's adventures. They co-direct the Native Health Initiative and have four children (Nizhoni, Bah'Hozhooni, Shandiin and Sihasin) who are the center of their lives.

He is deeply influenced by Indigenous culture and worldview through his marriage and twenty years of life working for and with Indigenous communities. As a white person, he continued to unpack White Privilege and acknowledges the honor it is to share Indigenous concepts, stories and art in this book. His hope is to share what some of what he has learned with respect, honor and humility as an ally and advocate for these communities.

In terms of writing, Anthony considers this one of his medicines and a part of his identity as a healer. He brings writing into his clinical work as part of a patient's treatment plan and has begun teaching writing as a form of wellness and self-care to fellow healers. When the pandemic began, his writing evolved into the Writing to Heal project. While this book includes the 2020 pieces, the blog continues with weekly inspirational pieces – https://writingtoheal1.blogspot.com.

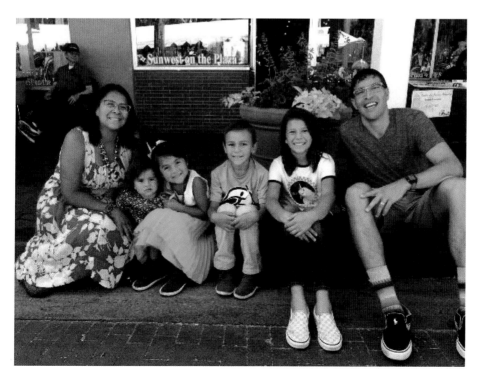

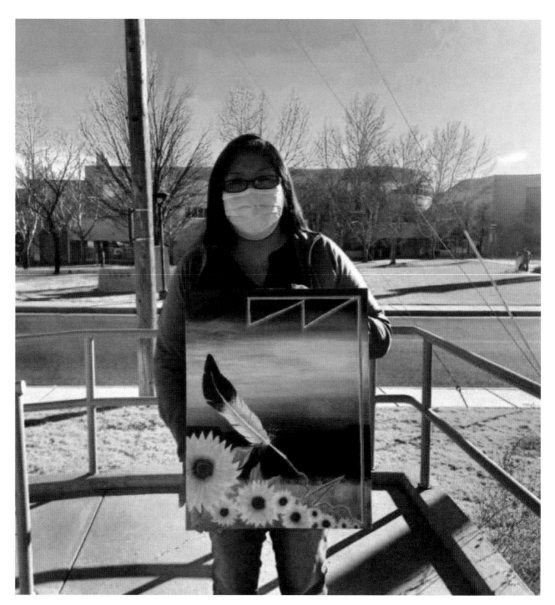

Cover Art by Mallery Quetawki

Mallery describes the work of art she created for the cover:

*Before the sky turns blue flooding the lands with light, a prayer is offered to the east at dawn. It is a prayer asking for the world to be wrapped in the safety of the ancestors, who now dance with the creator. Individuals who pray in the morning offer the same healing as those who are chosen healers, educated as providers and who truly bring care and comfort to our ailing neighbors. This particular morning prayer is for them. These healers of all shapes, sizes and disciplines carry the medicine deep within their heart, every beat counts, as it helps those around them bloom. May we all heal from things that hurt or haunt us and may we continue being good neighbors to one another. - **Mallery Quetawki***

Hand Font on front cover by **Jose "Chelo" Nunez**

Made in United States
Orlando, FL
14 February 2024

43691977R00058